REVERBERATIONS
A Daughter's Meditations on Alzheimer's

REVERBERATIONS

A Daughter's Meditations on Alzheimer's

Marion Agnew

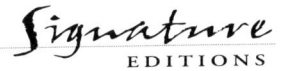

© 2019, Marion Agnew

All rights reserved. No part of this book may be reproduced, for any reason, by any means, without the permission of the publisher.

Cover design by Doowah Design.
Photo of author by Alan Dickson Photography.

This book was printed on Ancient Forest Friendly paper.
Printed and bound in Canada by Hignell Book Printing Inc.

We acknowledge the support of the Canada Council for the Arts and the Manitoba Arts Council for our publishing program.

Previous versions of these essays first appeared in the following journals:"Dripsody (Reprise)," Malahat Review; "Let d Be the Distance Between Us,"The Grief Diaries; "Words" and "All I Can Say," Room; "Backwards, Opposite, Contrary," Full Grown People; "Big Ideas, Small Feet" and "Hours of Daylight," Prairie Fire; "Fight Flight Freeze," NOWW Magazine; "Entanglement," Atticus Review; Nulliparous, Pithead Chapel; "Atomic Tangerine,"The New Quarterly.

Library and Archives Canada Cataloguing in Publication

Title: Reverberations : a daughter's meditations on Alzheimer's / Marion Agnew.

Names: Agnew, Marion, 1960- author.

Identifiers: Canadiana (print) 20190180323 | Canadiana (ebook) 20190180331 | ISBN 9781773240589 (softcover) | ISBN 9781773240596 (HTML)

Subjects: LCSH: Agnew, Marion, 1960-—Family. | LCSH: Agnew, Jeanne, 1917-2000—Health. | LCSH: Alzheimer's disease—Patients—Family relationships. | LCSH: Alzheimer's disease—Patients— Biography. | LCSH: Mothers and daughters. | LCGFT: Autobiographies.

Classification: LCC RC523.2 .A36 2019 | DDC 362.1968/3110092—dc23

Signature Editions
P.O. Box 206, RPO Corydon, Winnipeg, Manitoba, R3M 3S7
www.signature-editions.com

Contents

1	Dripsody (Reprise)	7
2	Let d Be the Distance Between Us	13
3	Polar Bears and Penguins	21
4	Words	31
5	Transitions: a Coding Secret	48
6	Backwards, Opposite, Contrary	51
7	Hours of Daylight (I)	61
8	The Tennessee Waltz	77
9	Meander (original title: Home)	86
10	All I Can Say	95
11	The House That Broke My Heart	102
12	Saguaro	113
13	Fight Flight Freeze	126
14	Big Ideas, Small Feet	133
15	Driftglass	141
16	Entanglement	147
17	Nulliparous	156
18	Atomic Tangerine	170
19	Hours of Daylight (II)	183
20	Reverberations	186

1

DRIPSODY (REPRISE)

Tick, tick. Tuck. Tick-tick.
The rain taps on the roof, an irregular metronome measuring years. It's August of 1992, and the chilly, damp morning makes for a smoky fire in the kitchen's wood-burning stove. My sister Sue and I crowd close anyway, fingers curled around coffee mugs. We're up early, determined that the weather won't spoil our summer vacation at our family camp just two dozen yards away from Lake Superior.

Though some "camps" are equivalent to "cottages," our camps are far less grand. In 1924, the summer my mother turned seven, my grandfather built a basic timber-framed rectangle, with a stone fireplace in one corner and a stove made from a fifty-gallon drum. In the 1930s, he extended the rectangle to create bedrooms. He "remodelled" its kitchen for Mom in the late 1940s, when she married and thought of children, by extending the concrete slab floor and adding more shelves.

Over the years, my grandparents accumulated ten acres along the shore. In the 1950s, my grandfather built a second camp on a different beach at the other end of the property. Mom had electricity and indoor plumbing added in the 1980s. Our parents stay in the second camp, out of sight but hardly out of mind.

My sister and I prefer what we laughingly refer to as the "rustic charm" of the original camp. The alterations in the intervening fifty years haven't changed its essential nature. Above us, no ceiling, only the underside of the roof—one-by-six boards covered in tarpaper and green pebbled roofing paper, sealed with tar—separates us from the weather.

A raindrop creeps down the stove's metal chimney. Another, driven between boards, splashes a hiss on the warm stovetop, a cymbal's brush accompanying the irregular mallet beat.

Tsss-sss. Tock. Tuck-tuck. Tick.

When I hear rain on a roof, I always think of summer vacations at this cottage. As a child, snugged into the flannelette-sheeted bed with Sue at night, I learned to distinguish between the patter of raindrops and the pitter of chipmunk feet on the roof. During the long summer days with our brothers, we sawed and split wood, swam and rowed, and, in the twilight, sang folk songs around the beach fire over which we'd just blistered hot dogs and torched marshmallows.

Even as my sister and I approach middle age, we feel free and happy here, and we try every year to pry ourselves away from the responsibilities of our lives and workplaces to spend time with our parents in this beloved place. Here, we're surrounded by childhood memories—not only ours, but our mother's, which she shares in stories featuring her brother, Hugh LeCaine.

* * *

Hugh Le Caine was a pioneer of twentieth-century electronic music. In 1955, at his laboratory at the National Research Council in Ottawa, he created the ninety-second piece "Dripsody" from an eye-dropper, water, a metal wastebasket, a microphone, and his experimental multi-track tape recorder. In his official biography by Gayle Young, *The Sackbut Blues*, he describes the creation of his most famous musical composition.

From a one-half-hour tape, the sound of a single drop was chosen.

The finished piece has been played for audiences in concert halls; it's been used in soundtracks for animated films. It's percussive and melodic, unpredictable and challenging, yet ultimately satisfying. And it all starts with a drop of water, recorded and re-recorded and manipulated into a coherent composition, a vehicle for a story.

* * *

When my mother and Uncle Hugh were children, he kept Mom entertained during family fishing vacations on Lake Superior by spinning tales about the family cat, who was really a Martian king in disguise. When my grandfather built the camp, the family used it as a summer home. At camp, Uncle Hugh and my mother played the way we did decades later—they swam, picked berries, built rafts, and raced snails on flat rocks.

Though she was three years younger, my mother was placed in his grammar school class. After they did homework, he'd disappear into the basement to work on science experiments. He was equally devoted to music. Once, the pianist for the church's play quit at the eleventh hour and Uncle Hugh stepped in to play the entire musical score, by ear, from memory. After they graduated from high school in the early 1930s, my grandmother moved heaven and earth, and the household, to ensure that both studied at Queen's University.

During the early days of the Second World War, each found government work in Ottawa. They roomed together but gravitated to opposite schedules. My mother, the early riser, kept house. She'd make a pumpkin pie, only to come home from work in the evening to find that my uncle, the night owl, had eaten the filling for "breakfast" before he left for his "day."

"Just the filling—of the whole pie!" she'd say, with a shake of her head and an indulgent laugh. "That made me so mad! What was I supposed to do with an empty piecrust?"

***

Some of the sounds had a wavering pitch which gave the drop a gurgling sound; others had pitch glides of over an octave. To simplify the problem of composition, the simplest and most formless sound was chosen, although the drops with complicated pitch changes were passed over with great regret.

***

Uncle Hugh didn't return to the camp after the early 1960s, when Grandma was in hospital. Mom says Hugh preferred to remember them—both the camp and their mother—as they had been in his childhood, vital and magical.

But he's always seemed particularly present to my mother here. This summer is no exception, and we hear many stories about him. Listening to the rain, Mom has said, "I know he made up 'Dripsody' to demonstrate one of his inventions, but I'm sure he thought to use a drop of water after hearing the rain on this roof."

In fact, Sue and I have noticed that Mom has begun repeating her childhood stories several times in the same day. We know that our grandmother, her mother, also repeated stories during the early stages of her decline into dementia. I wonder what, if anything, we should say to Mom. Although Sue and I are both aware of the repetition, we don't talk about it—a weak effort to pretend it isn't real. On that morning in 1992, the rain is an insistent tap on my shoulder, reminding me to worry. As if I could forget.

I wonder whether my mother worries, too. We can't gauge how Mom is aging by comparing her health to Uncle Hugh's. After a motorcycle accident, he died in 1977.

I look over at my sister, grateful for her companionship at that moment and, I hope, in the years ahead.

* * *

I chose the pentatonic scale to represent the order imposed on the pitch scheme by the listener. I don't believe that water actually drips in the pentatonic scale, but I believe that we tend to use our past hearing experience to organize a fresh collection of sounds that we hear.

* * *

Tip tuck tsss tip-tuck tuck-tip-tuck tsss-sss tuck-tuck.

That summer, my sister and I are unsure what we can do, what there even is to do, about our parents, about the camp. Our parents won't consider giving up control of the family property, and although we're adults, we can't afford to take it on. But the camp and our parents are aging. Someone will need to make decisions, and soon.

Meanwhile, Sue and I are suspended—between childhood stories and adult realities, between what's possible and what's inevitable, between what we know and what we don't, between what we try not to see before us and what we dread the future holds. We clutch our coffee mugs and replenish the fire in the stove, talking of the ambitious breakfasts Mom cooked on the wood stove when we were kids—oatmeal with brown sugar, scrambled eggs, toast and honey, and hot chocolate.

The rain strengthens and changes timbre. Some drops sharpen while others become round, inherently humorous splats. Sue and I exchange smiles. A row of drops dangles at the roof seam between the kitchen and the main room. Some drips release there, onto the wood or the concrete floor, while others glide down a crossbeam before falling with a snap onto the linoleum counter.

Sue and I find metal saucepans and Melmac teacups to catch the drips. We're not sure why we bother. The line between "indoors" and "outdoors" here has always been porous. But Mom used to slide saucepans under drips during rainstorms when we were young, so we do, too.

And we laugh, as Mom often does while telling stories of Uncle Hugh. We laugh because crying about the fragility of the cottage roof, of our mother's health, won't help. We laugh because our memories are of childhood, and freedom, and we hope that continuing to laugh will help us carry joy into the future.

The drip-catchers' materials add still newer voices to the composition. We say, "It's 'Dripsody'!" and listen to the music.

2

LET d BE THE DISTANCE BETWEEN US

a = My Favourite Paper

I'm leaving my parents' house after staying with them for the Christmas holidays. My mother hugs and kisses me. "I'm so glad you came. After all, you're my favourite paper."

I beam. "Of course I am. And you're my favourite mother."

In recent days, my mother has turned to me with childlike trust when she feels overwhelmed by all the strangers in her house, strangers who are her own grown children and her young grandchildren. Her guard is down; she is vulnerable. At last, she needs me.

She has Alzheimer's disease.

b = What Did You Miss?

My mother was once *that* parent, the one who says, "What did you miss?" when the child scores 99 percent on a test. That happened to me, only it was a 97 in eighth-grade algebra.

It wasn't just tests, either. At age eight or even eighteen, I'd sit at the dining room table, hunched over my homework. My mother would pass through the room, and I'd cringe because I knew what was coming.

"How's your long division?" she'd ask—or perhaps it was algebra, geometry, trigonometry, or calculus.

"Oh, fine," I'd say. "Just finishing up." Then I'd sit back and try to close my notebook, but I was never quick enough.

"Let's see here," she'd say, standing behind me. And then it was over. The Teacher had appeared, and that meant The Daughter had become an Idiot.

She'd sigh. "Well, that one's not right. And the rest of these are all wrong, too. Look, first, you need to sharpen your pencil. I don't know how you can possibly think properly with a pencil that dull. Never mind erasing here, just start on a fresh piece of paper. Yes, start over completely. Now, why did you think this was the right way to begin? You're like my students, just copying what I write on the board without *really stopping* to *think*. I don't know how you're ever going to learn if you insist on doing that."

The notebook page would blur as my eyes filled. *I'll never get it right.*

Now I better understand what my mother explained then—that what I didn't know was important, that spotlighting what I missed is how homework or a test showed me what I still needed to learn. Even at the time, I understood this concept, intellectually.

But I also understand now, as I felt back then, that there's a lot to be said for celebrating what's right before focusing on what's wrong, for recognizing competence and achievement before searching out and analyzing mistakes.

c = What You Have to Do

Ever since I can remember, I've flipped through photos from my mother's childhood in an effort to know the woman beyond the Mom who so dominated my early life.

I've tried to imagine what life was like when my mother was the little girl in bloomers and woollen stockings with a hole at the knee, delightedly cuddling a newly hatched seagull.

The brilliant young woman graduating with a university degree in mathematics in the late 1930s, listening with her father and sister to war news on the radio.

The glowing newlywed, reunited at the end of the Second World War with her naval officer husband after a few weeks together and then twenty-seven months apart.

The new mother whose first baby died the day it was born, who handled her grief by taking a teaching job the next week.

These women in my mother lived before I was born. Each continued to live, frozen inside white borders and secured between thick black sheets of scrapbook paper, but her experiences had long been assimilated into the composite woman, the Mom I knew. The woman who taught graduate students and pursued her own research interests, ran a strict household, and raised my four siblings and me.

When I'd find a photo of something from my mother's life that I thought might bring up a sad or difficult memory—perhaps a picture of Grandma in her later years—I'd linger over it. How would Mom see this picture? When I felt particularly brave, I'd show it to her, and she'd tell a story of her mother's dementia, of clearing out their family home, of Grandma's funeral.

I'd ask, "Were you afraid? Was it hard for you?"

She'd think for a moment. "Well, you just do what you have to do. Then you go on."

Yes, okay, I would think. *But was it hard? Were you afraid?*

$$d = My\ Darling\ Girl$$

My grandmother called my mother "my darling girl," but my grandmother also developed dementia. By the time my mother was in her early forties, Grandma no longer knew who she was.

I was in my late thirties when my mother's diagnosis came—a grown woman, as my mother had been—but not old enough. Then again, perhaps no age would be old enough.

e = Write Down What You Know

Not every homework session ended with me in tears. She taught me how to approach "word problems," those difficult scenarios that made you apply concepts.

"Start by writing down what you know," she'd say. "A train is travelling at an average of 60 miles per hour. That means the speed—call it s—is equal to 60. Write that down."

I'd write $s = 60$.

"Another way to say it is 'Let s equal 60.' You might see that in other problems. Okay, now look at what else this says. It takes 5 hours for the train to go from one town to the other. And that means…?"

With a little more prompting, I'd let t be the time—5 hours. So $t = 5$. And I could read that what we wanted to know—x—was how far apart the towns were. Using s and t, the speed and time, I could solve for x.

"We use x generally to mean something we don't know," Mom pointed out. "In this case, you could also call it d, for distance."

Little by little, I learned to see how mathematical symbols could replace English to represent what happened in the problem. A translation, of a sort.

"It's all in how you set up the problem," Mom would say. "After you get it set up correctly, the rest is just work."

It's taken me many decades to understand a little of her symbols, her language. Now I try to remember that her nagging came from her belief that I could do anything and everything, even though she never just said so. Instead, she showed me the distance I had yet to go—not the distance I'd come.

f = The Meanest Mom Ever

One day when I was in junior high, I was talking with a friend about a substitute teacher. "She's really mean," I said. "I sure would hate it if she were my mother."

My friend turned to me in surprise. "Oh, *we* all think *your* mother is the meanest mom *ever*."

I flushed with shame. "Meaner than this teacher?" I knew the answer but couldn't believe it until I heard it.

"Oh, yeah," said my friend with cheerful sympathy. "We don't know how you stand it."

I didn't know what to say. She was my mother, so of course I loved her, however "mean" she seemed, however much I might not *like* her in any particular moment. I never found a way to explain that. Or defend her, for that matter.

g = Egg Whites + Sugar

I know in my head that my mother has Alzheimer's disease, but somehow I'm still surprised, and my heart hurts, when I see these changes in the take-charge woman she used to be.

Earlier during those Christmas holidays, I'd noticed that she doesn't understand the words she's reading aloud.

"Mare-in-gyoo," says the woman who studied French for years, looking at *meringue* on a menu. Suspicion curls her upper lip. "Well, I don't know about *that*," she huffs, as if eggs whites and sugar are conspiring against her.

She can't follow a recipe. They have too many steps, and she gets sidetracked while cooking. She can't follow the thread of a narrative, so she can't lose herself in her beloved mystery novels. She needs to be entertained, as a young child does, because her own thoughts can't keep her company anymore.

At our weekly phone calls, I have to add, "This is your younger daughter" after I say my name, to try to make my abstract presence more real to her.

Those tiresome "stages of grief," though applied far beyond their original context, remain my familiars. Sometimes I feel them all at once. Anger at the disease, the horror of it. Denial that Mom has moved abruptly from "mild" to "moderate" Alzheimer's and requires more care than my eighty-one-year-old father can give, though he won't accept help. Bargaining that if I do the right things, if I can just channel some magic, she'll get well. Depression, at imagining life without her, which congeals into a stark, black envy at seeing two or three generations of mothers and daughters, talking together.

And fleeting moments of acceptance, when I can see the changes in my relationship with my mother as a reprieve—not by any means a "gift," but a chance to close a little of the distance between us.

Because at last, her expectations of me have changed. It's enough, for her, that I'm there with her at the holidays, helping her plan and put together meals, my familiar face helping smooth her interactions with our extended family.

$$h = Solve\ for\ x$$

The Christmas holiday when I am christened her "favourite paper" serves as a beginning, of a sort. Throughout the next months, as Mom continues to change, I try ever harder to stay connected to her. The concept of email is incomprehensible to my parents; however, they appreciate receiving mail. My father reads letters to her after supper. It's a highlight of their day.

And so almost every day, I mail an inane note: "Dear Mommy, I saw two pelicans on my way to work today. I didn't know they lived in the middle of Colorado. They were on the pond where I've seen the duck family."

The trivial and mundane are now the substance of our communication. I hope that by babbling about my own genuine delight in sunny days, beautiful snowfalls, and mountains that appear from behind clouds as if by magic, I can share her return to a life of "this moment." A form of childhood.

Our phone conversations stretch my imagination, because I can't rely on her words. She'll say, "We have the most beautiful picters, one over…by the, at the, there, and the other a good ways, maybe, oh, half a one, or a three, a third of the way down the octer, and it has one, two, three on it."

Solve for x. It helps that I visited at Christmas. "Three blooms on the begonia, in front of the window? That's great, Mom; you must be taking good care of it. And the geranium, by the door—how is it doing?"

As time passes, I have to listen even more carefully. I mentally stand where she is in the house, trying to see what she's pointing at. A new picture by the clock? New placemats on the table? Is it something that's really new, or something that simply caught her attention at that moment?

I search the tones of her voice for clues—sadness or worry or pleasure. Although she almost always has trouble with nouns, sometimes she can still pull out entire coherent phrases or sentences, usually social niceties. "It's good to see you." "I enjoy talking with you." "That's just great."

"And what are you doing these days?" she sometimes asks.

Oh boy, today is a good day. "Well, I work at a publishing company, editing books. They're kind of like the ones you wrote on number theory and linear algebra." Our conversation feels stilted, but I can't help myself. I want to remind her of who she was, to see if anything triggers memories or even just enjoyment.

She responds, "Oh, and I expect you're good at that."

I smile. A compliment! "You know how it is, Mom, they never turn out the way I want them to. I always see something I could have done differently."

She laughs. *Laughs!* "Well, I've been trying to, like that, for, a long time. I…it's…." She wants to say more but can't seem to get started.

I help her. "I know, I know—when I figure out how to make it perfect the first time, I'll give you a call."

Amusement bubbles in her voice. "Yes, thanks, you do that," she answers.

Sometimes, of course, I can't decipher her meaning (*let* d *be the distance between us*) and we're both frustrated.

But always when we end the conversation, she says, "We'll have to get together soon, and I'll enjoy that a lot," and I bless those phrases that remain. I try to remember that the love stretching between us isn't as tenuous as our ability to express it.

I admire her courage in staying on the phone, valiantly trying to participate in a conversation she can't fully follow, to be with people she knows must belong to her somehow.

i = It's Just Work

After I hang up the phone, I let the tears come—for all of the women she's been, the ones I've known and the ones I didn't get to meet.

Sometimes I even wish for math homework, just so she could teach me again.

I also want to thank her, though I'm not sure exactly what for—for believing in me, in her own way? For being the meanest mom *ever*? For telling me that I'm her favourite paper?

Those last thoughts make me laugh, but then the knot in the pit of my stomach grows again. There's so much ahead that I don't know how to handle.

So, I'll start by writing down what I *do* know. Maybe then I'll be able to frame the problem correctly. After that, it's just work, and I'll do what I have to do—accept even more changes in my mother, until all the women she ever has been exist only in photos and in memories. Solve for *d*, the distance between us, for as long as I can.

3

POLAR BEARS AND PENGUINS

Dad turns off the car and Mom looks back at us from the front seat. "Now, you five stay in the car, and no fighting. Lee's in charge. We'll be back to get you in a few minutes, and you'll come in and see Grandma. Decide what you want to sing. Sue, make sure Marion brings her book."

I peer over the back seat from the rear of the station wagon. The dark blue belt on Mom's dress is the same colour as the car seats. Dad puts his hand on Mom's back as they walk up the steps of a big, red-brick building. The boys pull out books, and Sue is drawing. Pete hums "Puff the Magic Dragon."

When our parents are out of sight, Lee gets out of the back seat and opens the front passenger door. "Shove over."

Hugh scoots across the slippery fabric till he's behind the wheel. He cranks down the window. Lee sits in Mom's place and leaves his door open to catch the breeze. Pete and Sue have their windows down, too.

The floor is hard back here in the tail. When we drive to Canada from Oklahoma for our summer vacation, I ride back here on top of the sleeping bags and pillows, squeezed beside the suitcases and ice chest and picnic basket. But yesterday, we unloaded the car at camp and now the pillows and sleeping bags are spread on our cots. So I'm sitting on the hard floor.

I say to Sue in the back seat, "Can I sit by you?" She sighs. "Okay, but you have to sit still."

I swing my legs over the back of the seat and slide down to stand on the seat.

"Quit bouncing," Pete says.

I let my legs buckle and sit with a plop.

He is mean, as usual. "I said, quit bouncing."

"I wasn't, I was sitting." I turn to Sue. "What are you doing?"

"Drawing." Her forehead wrinkles as her pencil moves across the page.

"Can I see?" Sometimes she makes books for me.

"No. Maybe later."

It's hot. I'm bored.

Hugh says from the front seat, "I wish we didn't have to come to town on our first day here."

Pete echoes, "Yeah, I want to go swimming."

I say to Sue, "What are we doing?"

"We're visiting Grandma. She's sick." She blows a little air out her lower lip to cool her face. I try it, and it ruffles my bangs.

"Do you think we'll come every day?" asks Hugh. He rests his chin on the back of the front seat. His chin pushes his whole head up and down when he talks.

"Probably," says Sue. "We always do." She sounds like she's mad, but I don't know why. I didn't do anything.

"We do?" I say.

"You're just a baby. No wonder you don't remember," Pete says.

"Am not! I'm four!"

Lee looks back. "So what are we singing? If I had my guitar we could do 'Blowin' in the Wind.'" He pushes his glasses up his nose.

"*Sound of Music.*" Sue sounds like Mom. Lee's the oldest, but Sue's the boss.

"We did that last year," says Hugh.

"So? Grandma won't remember." Sue still sounds mad. I look up, but she's looking at her page. Her pencil makes a *sh-sh-sh-sh* noise.

"She might," Lee offers. "She used to write me letters."

Sue sighs. "Ten years ago."

I quit listening. I kick my saddle shoes against the blue-carpeted hump of the floor of the car. My feet thud against the floor and click when my shoes hit each other. *Thud, click, thud, click.*

"Cut it out. Don't be a brat," says Sue.

I fold my arms across my lap.

"Bratty Marion," sings Pete.

Hugh puts his face to his open window. "Ahh, a breeze!"

I stand on the hump and grab the back of the front seat, trying to feel air moving.

Lee says, "Hey, quit it." He whacks my hands with his paperback book until my fingers let go of the cloth and I fall back, half on top of Sue.

"Look what you made me do!" She flashes her paper at me, but my tears make it blurry.

"Quit crying, you brat." Pete pulls me upright on the seat.

Sue's words are short. "Just—just get in the back."

"But it's hot." I climb over the seat into the tail again. My foot bangs Pete accidentally on purpose and he grabs it.

"Now *you* cut it out," Sue tells him.

He lets go. "You're not the boss of me."

I slump in the tail. My shoes make a different sound on this floor. There's no carpet, so they thunk instead of thudding. *Thunk thunk thunk thunk.*

"Quit kicking. Here." Sue hands a book over the seat. "Read this."

"I don't know how."

"You know how it goes."

The book is about penguins and polar bears. I do know how it goes. I turn pages, whispering the story. The pictures are black and white, except for the penguins' orange beaks and the blue water.

"Here comes Dad," Lee says.

Everybody starts rolling up windows. Clutching my book, I try to climb out over the seat, but it's full of elbows and knees.

Pete is tying his shoes. "Would you just wait?"

Finally, they're all out. I slide down the back of the seat, bouncing as I land. I climb out of the car.

Sue asks, "Where's your book?"

I show it to her. She brushes at my short hair with her fingers and slaps at my rumpled corduroy pants to straighten them.

"No wonder you're hot, in those pants. Why did you wear them?"

I look down and back up at her, surprised she has to ask. "'Cause they're my favourite, 'cause…"

Pete says mockingly with me, "There's pockets in 'em, that's why."

"Yep," I say. Out of the car, the breeze feels good. I can't see Lake Superior from here, but the air feels like it visited the lake before it got to me. White birch trees stand tall in groups in the flat green lawn. I want to run, but Sue grips my hand. We all walk to the building.

"Dad," says Lee, "is Grandma in bed, or is she still in an apartment?"

Dad turns to him. "She's in a large room now, without a kitchen. But we'll visit in the parlour. Now, children." He stops on the steps. "You need to be on your best behaviour. You're representing the family, and this is very important to your mother."

"Yes, sir," we chorus.

Then Pete asks, "Will Grandma remember us?"

Dad says slowly, "She always loves to see children, and she'll be very glad to see you."

The five of us file into the building ahead of Dad. Inside, it's dim. Echoes of our footsteps shoot along the polished floors of three different hallways. It smells kind of like the outhouse at camp. I close off my nose from inside and breathe through my mouth.

"This way," Dad says. We go down a long hallway and turn into a big, bright room. I run to Mom where she sits on the couch. She's talking to an old lady who sits in the chair beside the couch, in front of a tall window. Other couches and chairs face each other in groups around the room, and other people are sitting in them.

"Well, hello," says the old lady in a high voice, smiling.

"This is Marion," Mom says. "Say hello, Marion." The lady's white hair stands up all around her face like rays from the sun. I look away, my finger in my mouth.

"This one's shy." Mom's voice is sad.

I look back to see if the lady is still looking at me. She's smiling and nodding at the others as they say, "Hi, Grandma." But she could look at me. I know she could. My stomach hurts. I hide my face in Mom's lap.

Mom pulls me up to sit on the couch beside her. I put my book in front of my face, but Mom puts it in my lap. Holding my arms down, she whispers, cross like she is in church, "Sit up straight and be-*have*." I sit still.

Mom says to Sue, "What are you singing?"

The lady says, "They're singing? Lovely." She leans forward in her chair.

Sue says, "'My Favourite Things.'"

I don't sing on this one. The others stand in front of the couch in a big curve, like when Lee skips a rock over the water. They line up by height and age: Lee, Sue, Hugh, Pete. Fifteen, thirteen, eleven, and nine. Sue picks a note and they start.

My shoes tap together in time to the singing. *Tip tap tap tip.* Mom puts her hand on my leg and shakes her head at me. I quit tapping and look at the lady. Grandma. Her face is tall, not round. Her teeth are big when she smiles.

They are singing, "Snowflakes that stay on my nose and eye-LASH-es…."

I lean back against the couch and look up at Mom. She's watching Grandma. Mom's lower lip wobbles. I scoot closer and she puts her arm around me.

They're at Pete's favourite part: "When the DOG BITES, when the BEE STINGS…" He likes to shout and say "sting" like "stink," but this time he doesn't. His head is down. Hugh stares ahead, like he's looking out a window, but Sue and Lee look at Grandma. Lee's Adam's apple bobs and he smiles as he sings.

Pete looks up for the end, "I don't feeeeeeeel…so baaaaaad." They bow as Grandma claps. Other people in the room clap, too.

A lady in a white outfit with a white cap walks by and smiles at us. She stops and says, "Mrs. LeCaine, you have visitors! Are these your grandchildren?"

Mom's arm tightens around me. Grandma answers, "Grandchildren? Why, I don't—"

Dad speaks up. "Yes, we're family, visiting from Oklahoma."

"How nice," says the white lady. She walks away.

Mom says, next to my ear, "Ask Grandma to read your book to you."

My insides go cold. I look at Mom and shake my head.

Mom's eyebrows are black across her face and her ice-blue eyes snap. "Go." She picks me up under my arms and swings me to the floor. Pete slides behind me to sit in my spot, giving me another shove.

One hand on Mom's knee, I walk around her toward Grandma.

Grandma motions toward the book. "Would you like to do this?" Her voice is high and crackly.

I nod, still holding Mom's knee.

"Well, come here, then." She leans forward and I stand beside her chair, where I can see the pictures. Grandma takes the book.

"You hold this side, and I'll hold this other one. Oh, this is a nice one. See here, bears and birds." She opens the cover.

I say, "They're polar bears and penguins."

Her voice smiles at me. "Yes, they are, aren't they? Now, let's see here, what does this fellow do? He lies there, that's all. And this one? He's not so lazy."

I frown. This isn't how the story goes. I whisper, "They're happy and playing." That's what happens on that page.

"What's that?" asks Grandma.

I say it louder. "They're happy and playing."

"Yes, it looks like they are. What about this side, these fellows?"

I don't say anything. Am I supposed to keep telling her the right story? But I'm not supposed to talk back to grownups. I'm not sure how to stay out of trouble.

Grandma says, "Well, these fellows look good to me, too. Let's see what happens next."

I turn over the page for Grandma to hold. She puts her arm around me. I lean on the flat wooden arm of her chair.

"Oh, look. Now they're swimming. Doesn't that water look cold? I think this guy says to that one, 'It's too cold to go in. I'm staying out here where it's warm.' Do you think he would say that?"

I bob my head up and down once. That's not what the bear really says, but he could. But everybody else knows that's not what the bear says. I'm waiting for Pete to say something mean.

I peek over at him and Mom. She dabs at her eyes with a Kleenex that has red lipstick spots on it.

Grandma says, "I think this guy is sleepy, so he naps while the other guy swims."

This is all wrong. But the picture does look like that. And then for each page, Grandma tells a whole new story about the bears and penguins. Her hands holding the book look like Mom's, with blue rivers standing up under the skin. Her thumb is wide and square.

We get to the last page. "And the friends were very happy," says Grandma. "Wouldn't you be?"

I look up at her.

"The end." She hugs me a little. I let her, and then I take the book back.

"What lovely trousers you have on."

"They're my pumpkin-coloured pants with pockets in 'em, that's why." She laughs. I slip back to stand by Mom's knee.

"What do you say, Marion?" Mom's voice is her teacher-voice.

"Thank you, Grandma." I wiggle to stand between Pete's legs and Mom's.

"You're welcome," she says.

"Hey, Grandma," Lee puts in. "I'm almost an Eagle Scout!"

"Oh, lovely," says Grandma. "Are you working hard at it?"

Grandma and Lee talk more while I think about my book. Grandma told me a story about pictures that used to tell another story. It puzzles me.

Then Grandma turns to Mom and says, "Well, it's been delightful, but I have a meeting and must be going." She stands up.

Mom says, "Can't you stay for another song?"

Grandma's forehead wrinkles. "Oh, I don't know."

"Just one." Mom shoots Sue and Lee a look. They stand up.

Grandma says, "Well..."

Mom puts her hand on Grandma's arm. "A short one."

Grandma smiles at her. "All right then, thank you." She sits, and Mom pats her arm.

The four of them line up again, and Sue motions to me, too. I stand in front of her and she puts her hands on my shoulders, then she picks a note and starts singing. "Let's start at the very beginning, a very good place to start. When you read, you begin with..."

"A, B, C," I say loudly. Pete says it with me. Some people behind us laugh. Sue goes on, "When you sing, you begin with do, re, mi..."

My part is over. She pushes me toward Mom, who holds out her hands. I stand between her and Grandma.

While they sing the rest of "Doe a Deer," I watch Grandma. Her hands are folded in her lap and they clap a little in rhythm. At the end, everybody claps again.

The lady in the white outfit is clapping too. Next to her is a man in a blue suit. She says to the man, "These people are Mrs. LeCaine's family, from the States."

Mom and Dad stand up and shake hands with the man. "I'm her daughter, Jeanne." Grandma has stood up, too. She says,

"Daughter? Haven't seen her in ages." She turns to Mom. "It's been a delightful visit, but I have a meeting and must be going."

The white lady puts her hand under Grandma's arm. "Let's find the washroom, shall we?"

As they walk away, Mom calls out, "See you tomorrow, Mother." Grandma doesn't turn around. I look up at Mom. She never cries, but her eyes are full of tears, and she blows her nose.

Sue takes my hand. "Come on, we're going outside."

As the five of us pass the grownups, the man says, "...very normal at this stage..." and Mom nods, Kleenex over her nose.

Once we're outside, Sue lets go of my hand and I run to the green grass. I turn a somersault and then lie looking at the blue sky and the green birch leaves before I sit up and look around.

Sue sits on the steps of the building. She blows her nose.

I go lean on her knees. "What's wrong?"

More tears come down her face. I sit down close beside her on the step. She says, "Wouldn't it be terrible if Mom didn't know who you were?"

I don't understand. She's Mom. How could she not know me?

"Like when she's mad and won't talk to you. Only forever." She folds her arms across her knees and puts her head down. I don't like it when Sue cries. My eyes fill with tears.

Then Mom and Dad come out.

"Here, what's this?" Dad's voice isn't quite jolly, but he's not mad.

Sue wipes her face and we get up. "Nothing."

Mom's nose is red, and her mouth is still trembly. She takes my hand and hugs Sue with her other arm, not saying anything. We walk to the car, where the boys are waiting.

On the way home, I'm in the front seat between Mom and Dad. The car sways gently as Dad takes the curves of the highway. I put my head on Mom's lap. My eyes keep closing.

Mom rubs my back gently. "She never did read the story that was in the book."

"No, she never did," Dad says. "She loves seeing the kids."

"Yes. Even if she doesn't know them. Or me." Mom sighs. "I expected it. But still."

"She looks healthy."

"Yes, she thinks she still has meetings."

Mom sounds very far away. The polar bear says to me, "I'm going swimming. Do you want to stay there where it's warm?"

4

WORDS

In mid-December, 1997, I stood at my kitchen table, flipping through the mail. Among the bills and ads, I found a couple of Christmas cards.

"Hey, this one's from Mom," I said aloud. The card showed a sprig of mistletoe tied with a red ribbon. Under the printed greeting inside, Mom had signed "Jeanne" instead of her usual "Mother," and Dad had written, "Come see us! Ted." On the opposite page, Mom had written a note. As I read it, my stomach tightened.

> *I wish I had a time to visit together your during the avation. I enjoy very much some of the value evated as she sees us all. We enjoy very muh. I wish that all those precess that seem to have great help. Reap and the children are looking fast. Our children can "take forst" but we are working like greeting trying to see you again soon!*

I winced. When did she get this bad?

For ten months, since Mom's diagnosis the previous February, I'd had a name for her forgetfulness and confusion, her lost and mangled words. Until then, my sister and I had simply called it "how she is," as in "you know how she is." But even after her diagnosis, I'd allowed "probable Alzheimer's disease" to remain an abstraction, separate from the woman who was my mother.

This Christmas card, trembling slightly in my hand, showed me her disease—right here, blue ink on white paper.

I sagged into a chair, blinking away tears to examine the card. She had really worked at this note, adding the word "your" to the first sentence: "I wish I had a time to visit together *your* during the avation." Did it make sense to her then?

As I looked, my initial horror became embarrassment. My father had no memory problems—why had he let her send this? Why had he let her *expose* herself in this way? My embarrassment turned into annoyance at him, at his illegible scrawl. I looked again at what he'd written: "Come see us!"

Then I heard him—really heard him. *Come see us.* It was neither a command nor a demand; they were not his style. It was a plea beamed into the universe: "Is anyone there? Can anyone help us?" I felt the 800 miles between my home and theirs and sputtered sudden, guilty tears.

Most people think Alzheimer's disease is the same as memory loss. Well, *most* people don't think about Alzheimer's at all, if they can help it. Perhaps if we all ignore it hard enough, it will go away.

That was certainly my hope, even after I knew my mother's diagnosis. After all, I was still young, just in my thirties, with my own life concerns. My parents, who had been in their early forties when I was born, had always been satisfactory support for each other, their lives highly structured and extremely private. My four siblings and I had never spoken seriously and specifically with them about their money (that would be vulgar) or their health (that would be impertinent). Doing something active in relation to my mother's forgetfulness and agitation felt unthinkable, impossible. On the rare occasions I let myself wonder about her health, I wanted to go to bed and pull the covers over my head.

But now, I had to think about this disease. Learn about it.

As Mom walked down the path of her disease, words dropped behind her—names here, a noun there. The farther into the disease she went, the more quickly the words disappeared, swirling behind her like autumn leaves caught in a strong wind. So I took that as my starting point: words. As Mom lost them, I would learn new ones.

After the holidays, I finally forced myself to read her physician's diagnostic report from the previous year, which my father had shared with my siblings and me.

> *Patient has some problems with verbal communication, but no aphasia or paraphasias are noted. She did have some apraxia.... Mini-mental status examination reveals a dismal score of 5/30.*

From the dictionary, I learned that *aphasia* is a general inability to understand words and that *paraphasia* is the substitution of inappropriate words when speaking. *Apraxia* meant that Mom couldn't complete complex coordinated movements easily.

I already knew the meaning of the word *dismal*.

So, no aphasia or paraphasia? The assessment contradicted Mom's Christmas note. Still, I had noticed that she could still speak relatively well at the social level: "Hi, how are you; good to see you" were all phrases still close to the surface for her. Maybe the neurologist hadn't pushed the conversation beyond that level.

Or maybe Mom's abilities had deteriorated significantly in the year since this assessment.

Dismal.

> *On further neuropsychological testing, the patient failed in all major areas. She did very poorly on orientation, very poorly on attention. She could not do calculation very well but this was actually better than most other areas.*

My mother began school in Grade 2 and was moved to Grade 3 within weeks. Born Jeanne LeCaine in Port Arthur (now Thunder Bay), Ontario, Canada in 1917, she graduated from high school at fifteen. At Queens University, she graduated with a B.A. and an M.A. in mathematics and economics after four years. In 1938, she entered Radcliffe—the part of Harvard University open to women at that time—where she earned her Ph.D. in mathematics in 1941. During the Second World War, she worked in Ottawa and Montreal, researching neutron transport equations as part of Canada's atomic research project. After the war, she declined an invitation to move to Los Alamos, New Mexico, to continue nuclear research. She'd already married my father, a historian. Instead, she raised a family of five and became a university professor. During her career, she forged partnerships with mathematicians in industry and taught generations of mathematicians and future teachers.

This neuropsychological test, which my mother took at the age of seventy-nine, may have been one of the few tests she ever failed.

After reading the diagnostic report, I knew what to do next: research. My professor parents had trained me well.

I learned that memory is only one of the losses in people with Alzheimer's. In fact, "loss" is the overarching theme. Early in the disease, patients lose their car in the parking lot or lose track of what they meant to say. Later, they lose their roles in life: husband? daughter? parent?

At the end, they lose motivation. Awareness of their surroundings. Consciousness.

At that time, a positive diagnosis of Alzheimer's required an analysis of brain tissue. In other words, an *autopsy*.

So Mom's neurologist estimated. According to his calculations, my mother had been lurking in the early stages of the disease (confusion, some word loss) for some seven years. Recently, she had slid into the middle stage, with its *sundowning* (night wakefulness), *wandering* (compulsive and anxious walking), and *rummaging* (obsessively searching for unknown items). Her confusion and antagonism would only increase.

I learned that as Mom's disease progressed, she would probably hallucinate. She would not only see and hear things that weren't there, her senses of taste and smell might become involved. We could expect only her sense of touch to remain relatively unchanged. Aside from a ceremonial hug and kiss at arrivals and departures, my family didn't touch much. But after my reading, I began putting my hand on her arm or shoulder every chance I got.

And I made more chances to see them. Before receiving that Christmas card, I'd visited my parents just twice a year. I saw them six times before the next Christmas holiday. Travelling the 800 miles between my home and theirs, even flying, chewed up most of a day each way. For each visit, I took a four- or five-day weekend and usually travelled alone or occasionally with Sue, my sister.

Fortunately, my boss was very understanding. I used all my vacation days, my "personal days," and even sick leave for days I went to doctor's appointments with them. Difficult as these visits were, there was nowhere else I would have gone, nowhere else I would rather have been.

In early 1998, as Mom's disease moved into its middle stage, she began *wandering*—a common Alzheimer's symptom with a strikingly inaccurate name. Usually someone wandering meanders, drifts aimlessly from here to there. A person with Alzheimer's who wanders instead walks with a purpose.

In the spring, Mom's wandering increased. At least once a week, she slipped out of the house when Dad was inattentive for even a moment. Friends would see her five miles away and bring her home.

In other families, coping with illness may be less daunting than it was in ours. Mom's illness challenged our family's inertia, our unwillingness to believe she was failing. Other families may respond better to the "Can't you just..." questions. Can't you just move your parents here? Can't you just move there? Can't you just find a residence for her there? No, no, and no, not at that time. Solutions are easy to offer to other people's parents.

That spring, Dad and I talked on the phone every week. I squeezed my eyes tight as I listened to his historian's detailed description of their routine. Mom's wandering and belligerence pushed at his limits. She could not be alone, and neither could he. She was demanding, he was frustrated, and I couldn't help. For one thing, uprooting my life to be closer was impossible; my marriage, already not strong, would not survive. For another, even if I moved in with them, what could I do?

I focused on her wandering. I recognized her route—through the university campus to the highway leading toward I-35—as the beginning of our summer trip. The interstate would take her north to Duluth. From there, Highway 61 led to the Canadian border, Thunder Bay, and her home twenty miles beyond. To the camps at the lake.

I believed she was trying to get *home*—where she'd always felt most herself. So I resolved that Mom would go to the lake as usual in the summer. I was convinced she'd be happy there. As I talked with my sister about the trip, I'd say, "Of course, being there won't make her *well*." But inside me, a small voice whispered, *Anything can happen. You never know.*

I opened the camps in early July. Our handyman did the heavy work of removing shutters and setting up the water lines. I worked inside, sweeping out squirrel and mouse nests, stocking the refrigerator, and freezing a few meals for Dad to reheat after I left. I opened windows and trimmed branches to let in light and air.

Mom and Dad arrived in time for a late supper. We sat at a table overlooking the lake. My father reported, "So after our Memphis leg, we had three hours in Minneapolis, and we decided to get something to eat." He speared green beans on his fork and chewed them slowly.

Mom broke in, "Look, here comes another woman, swoop, down." She waved her empty fork in an arc, following a gull's flight.

I peered out at the water. "There's lots of gulls out there. They're pretty, aren't they?"

"So." Dad seized the floor. "We didn't go to the wicket at the International Terminal, the Hubert H. Humphrey Terminal, because I thought I remembered that they only had vending machines out there. But there's a central area in the main terminal with a TCBY, and a Starbucks, and a Lieutenant Colonel Somebody's fried chicken, and a Kinko's, and you can't eat there, but we kept walking along till we found something that looked good." He waited a moment before adding archly, "*Not* fried chicken."

I nodded. "That was smart of you to remember. That you couldn't get food out there, I mean."

Mom said, "Yes, it *was* good, and see now, there's a one, two, three, four, five. Oops, and here's another, six."

I looked out again. "Are you sure? I don't see that many."

Mom counted in a token whisper, pointing at each gull with her fork. "One, two, three."

Dad said, "So we found a sandwich place..."

"Four, five, and then a four..."

"Only we didn't *have* sandwiches, we had soup..."

"Six, seven..."

"And quiche and split it."

"Seven," Mom said more loudly. Another group of gulls circled and landed.

My turn. "Well, now there's more than seven, Mom," I said, adding to Dad, "What kind of quiche?"

"Hmmmm, let's see. Bacon and some kind of cheese. And was there onion, or was I just worried that there might be?" He put down his fork, pressed his right forefinger under his nose, and closed his eyes. The lines on his forehead and around his eyes smoothed slightly as he sat. His day had started twelve hours ago. Travelling is stressful when you're eighty-one, even when you're not caring for someone with Alzheimer's. I wondered just how hard this day had been for him.

My mother couldn't take her eyes off the gulls. "See, look, they just, whoops, away. Ups, and then no, they're back. So, one, two, three, no, I *got* that woman already, one, two—they don't stay *still* long enough for me to count them." Mom laughed, her white curls bobbing. I shared her delight.

"*No* onion." Dad opened his eyes again. "But some kind of sprouty things on the side." His wedding ring glowed golden in the early evening light as he waved his fingers to indicate sprouts.

"Eight," Mom said. "No, wait, no, just so—sev—seven."

"And tomato," he said brightly. "Cut up. Well, sliced."

"Ah. What kind of soup?" I turned to Mom. "Are you sure they don't go under to fish, and then come up again?"

"Well, yes, they might," Mom agreed. "In any case, it's lovely, and I'm glad to be here."

I smiled. *She understands where she is. She's glad to be here.*

She laughed. "Look, there's about a hundred—well, no, not *that* many, a five or so more."

Dad's eyes were still closed in contemplation of soup.

"Hey, look at that house out there." Mom pointed at Caribou Island glistening in the evening light. "It's got a lovely pink on it."

I seized the chance to get us all in the same conversation. "Hey, look, Dad; the sun is still shining out on Caribou."

He opened his eyes. "Broccoli cheese."

I sighed.

When I left to sleep at the other camp, my parents came outside to say good night. My mother said to me, "I've been here so much, I don't know whether I'm really here or just...thinking I am."

To hug her, I had to reach down. "You're really here." She leaned against me. We stood together in the midsummer twilight, looking out at the water, at Caribou floating in the dusk.

I stayed only a few days to ensure they were settled. About a week later, Dad said on the phone that he'd had to forestall Mom's demands to go "home" by driving into town. Back in Colorado, I hung up the phone and paced, desperately wanting him to be wrong. It just couldn't be true. She *was* home. I was sure she'd understood that. How could she not understand that?

Fearful and heartsick, I went to the lake again, just to see for myself.

My flight got in late. I stopped in at my parents' only to say hello before heading to the smaller camp to go to bed. Mom was happy to see me but sleepy and ready for bed. It was impossible to tell how she was from our brief conversation. We agreed that they'd follow our usual routine—they'd walk over to see me just before lunchtime.

The next morning, sunrise through the windows of our smaller camp woke me. I nestled in bed for a moment, watching the sunlight's pink and gold reflections dance on the ceiling, then sat up and stretched. The cool familiar smells, a combination of damp leaves and wood smoke, water and sunlight, cleared my head. *This is Mom's home. She must feel it. Dad must be wrong.*

As the sun began to climb the sky, I went for a leisurely row in the bay. The breeze welcomed me, circling the boat a few times before disappearing. Powerful and efficient, I skimmed across the water's surface.

I brewed coffee and took it down to the beach. When I heard a car pull up behind the camp, I checked my watch. A car? At 10:30?

Dad appeared around the camp's corner. He wore a sports coat and Hush Puppies, town clothes, instead of his usual camp attire, a moth-eaten cardigan, and tennis shoes.

"Good morning." I let my surprise register in my voice and face. "Where's Mom?"

"Right here." He sounded grim. She followed him around the camp, her mouth tight and her bright blue eyes narrowed. She too was dressed for town—a blouse and skirt with matching vest, clutching a handbag. Her hair was carefully brushed.

I stood up to kiss her. "Good morning, Mom."

She frowned. "He says he's taking me, but he's not." Disgust underlined her words.

"I beg your pardon?" I raised an eyebrow at Dad.

Mom's voice became cold and rough, her words short. "He's supposed to take me *home*." She held her purse in front of her with both hands.

Dad swept his arm like an emcee introducing an act. "This is how it works."

We stood in silence.

Stunned, I looked down at the mug I held. "How about a cup of coffee?"

"Well, if you must, I suppose." Her voice sounded flat, put-upon. She didn't move.

I led the way into the camp. Mom followed, scowling. Dad brought up the rear. I lit the propane burner and put water on for instant coffee. Mom sat down heavily in the rocking chair in front of the window and folded her hands over her purse.

I heard myself chattering. "It's been a gorgeous morning, hasn't it? Bright and sunny. When I flew in yesterday, we came across the bay from the south and the city lights along the shore were beautiful."

Dad stood in the kitchen with me, looking at his fingernails. Mom stared out the window, her mouth still tight. I swallowed and forced myself into silence.

When the coffee was ready, I carried a mug to Mom.

"Thank you." She took a sip. The harshness had disappeared from her voice, leaving it calm, even thoughtful. "Now, I'm looking at that one." She pointed out the window at a clump of trees—a perfectly formed balsam surrounded by a group of tall birches. "That one in the middle," she said, accenting her words with chopping motions. "Well, let's see, there's the stict one and the tocked one and then there's one that has legs just whoop, whoop, whoop, like that. And then the next ones are just...not." She took another sip of coffee.

Wary, I risked teasing her. "And I'm surprised you haven't demanded that we cut the branches off that tree. You always want a clear view of the water."

"Maybe so." Mom's eyes didn't waver from the trees.

Dad and I settled into chairs on either side of her. Bit by bit, I relaxed. The three of us drank coffee and chatted about nothing—the birds, the water, the birch trees.

Mom looked down at her watch. "Let's see, it's...why...it's time." She stood up. "Time to be...some, some food." She carried her mug into the kitchen.

"Huh." I checked my own watch. It was 11:45. I looked toward Dad.

He said, "We'll see you over at the other place for lunch in about a half hour."

"Sure." After they left, I stood in the kitchen. I pressed my palms into the linoleum countertop and bent my head. *She can't go home. She won't get well. Not even here. Not ever.*

After a trip, people always asked, "So did you have fun visiting your parents?"

The question stumped me. I didn't want to lie and just say "yes." I wanted everyone, everywhere to know that smart, capable people got Alzheimer's disease. I wanted everyone to know just a little of what my mother was going through, what it was like for my father and the family—but most people didn't *really* want to know. And I didn't want to embarrass either my mother or my father. I just wanted to tell some of the truth, but not so much that I drove people away.

Of course my visits weren't *fun*, not even according to my own parents' definition of fun activities—long conversations at the table after a meal, going to a college athletic event, working desultorily at a 1000-piece jigsaw puzzle as an excuse for more chatting, looking at family photo albums, singing at the piano. As Mom's abilities diminished, our activities changed. I picked small jigsaw puzzles that she could finish in about a half-hour, with my surreptitious help, to forestall her frustration and agitation. I spent a lot of time distracting Mom so that her constant, confused questions didn't send my father's understandable irritation over the edge into angry shouting, which upset all of us.

Throughout my visits, I blocked out the memory of the inquisitive, intelligent woman Mom had been to focus on who she still was: *Mom Now*.

I also couldn't think of these visits as the opposite of *fun*, whatever that might be. For one thing, they stretched ahead of me for the foreseeable future. And for another, beyond them lay only a future in which I didn't have even *Mom Now* to visit.

Eventually, I settled on another word: *rewarding*. "I had a rewarding time," I would say, adding, "Mom and I made cookies together." Or "Mom and I went shopping." Or "Mom and I were in the kitchen and she said she was glad I was there." *Rewarding* came to encompass everything I couldn't say.

While visiting my parents, I felt as if I were picking my way through a swamp at midnight, with dangers lurking in every direction.

Confronting some dangers required me only to grow up a little. I braved the family taboo on discussing money to learn that my parents' pensions adequately covered their expenses. I ventured gingerly into their health care by making lists of Mom's doctors and medications. After screwing up my courage, I asked to speak directly with my mother's doctors, even without her or my father present. My father wanted to give my mother good report cards, but the doctors needed to know what her abilities really were.

In fact, I found that confronting my father—gently but consistently—was the most dangerous and frightening part of this time. He was my mother's *caregiver*, a murky role that was very different from *husband*. He had never been skilled in the practical tasks of caring and comforting, and he lacked patience. He wouldn't accept that my mother couldn't learn and, in fact, would keep losing cognitive skills—her ability to focus on a book (and, later, to read), to distract herself from unhappy thoughts (later, to express them clearly), to watch an entire movie (later, to understand what she saw). She was not the woman he married, not the woman she'd become during their fifty years together.

She resisted bathing. She wore the same clothes, including underwear, day after day, and refused to discuss it with him. Worst of all, she couldn't recognize him as her husband. Some evenings she became scandalized, outraged at his expectation that she would sleep in their double bed. His response: shouting.

My father was angry: at the illness, at himself for not being able to cure her, at her for slipping away. He was angry at me for bearing witness to his short temper, for suggesting he comfort or indulge her when his inclination was to argue her "back to reality"—a trip she could not make. I was frightened of his anger, and I was plenty angry, too —angry that he wanted help and then wouldn't accept it. Angry that I wasn't doing enough, though I was doing all I could.

Aside from two extremely tense phone conversations, we didn't argue (that would have been vulgar) but we disagreed, and we knew we disagreed.

I kept reading—memoirs by caregivers, John Bayley's *Elegy for Iris*, memoirs by those in early-stage Alzheimer's. Nowhere could I find the book my father and I both needed so desperately—the one with the cure to my mother's illness, the one that would give her back to us.

Between Christmas of 1997 and April of 1999, simply watching the modulations of my mother's life gave everyday words a new texture and colour.

The obvious: *Inexorable, inevitable, erosion, diminish. Ambivalence*: After every visit, I hated yet was relieved to go.

Mixed blessing: Still having a mother to visit, but not the same mother I had known.

Bittersweet. Particularly when she and I, side-by-side in the middle of some simple activity, laughed together.

Sometimes *triumph, achievement.* My mother hummed the tunes as we watched an old musical together. My father had a nap while she and I chatted. At the breakfast table, she said she was delighted to see me.

Even *victory.* We made it through another day.

In April, 1999, my mother experienced seizures and spent a month in the hospital. The seizures, said the neurologist, marked her descent into the late stage of Alzheimer's. She lost the ability to act independently. Reminding her to eat drew only her impassive stare, but if fed, she'd eat with pleasure. Similarly, she could walk with a walker if she had a friendly, encouraging face backing up in front of her, but without it, she simply sat in a wheelchair.

She moved from the hospital into a nursing home just before Mother's Day, 1999. My sister, Sue, and I had timed our visit to help Mom adjust to the new routine. The day before, a tornado ripped through their region, flattening a small town. As the plane circled before landing, I saw what looked like light-grey confetti scattered across a red carpet. The confetti turned out to be metal and wood, pieces of a house that were now strewn across the raw, orange-red clay soil.

At the nursing home, Sue pulled our rental car into a parking spot and turned the key in the ignition. We didn't move. The late afternoon sun turned the humid air in the car into a sauna.

"Okay," I said more cheerfully than I felt, then bit my lip.

"We can do this," she said.

"Yes." I took a deep breath and let it out slowly. Silently, I repeated *We can do this, we can do this* as we reeled up and down halls where strong antiseptic couldn't quite cover the smell of human waste and fear. Televisions blared from some rooms; in others, residents moaned. Still others were silent and dark, the blinds drawn, the lumps under the sheets immobile.

Bewildered, we questioned everyone wearing scrubs until we pieced together the routine of bathing, clothing, hairdressing, feeding, exercising, laundering. Meanwhile, my mother sat in a wheelchair in her room, chin in hand.

Oh, the guilt at leaving her there, yet the relief that evening as Sue and my father and I shared a quiet meal at a restaurant. No more public wrangling of my mother's confusion and incoherent insistence for attention. No more makeshift dinners at home, one sister distracting Mom while the other foraged with my father. No more wakefulness, wondering if she was sneaking out of the house in a wandering fit. We let the professionals do the difficult parts of care for yet another version of *Mom Now*.

The biggest dangers in the walk through the nightmarish swamp were behind me. Gradually, the extra tension between my father and me dissipated. The journey—ours, hers—wasn't over, but we could continue as a united family.

My first day back at the office, a coworker asked whether my parents lived near the path of the tornado. "Did you see much destruction?" she said.

I thought of the woman I'd left frowning at a catalogue, trying to pick the printed flowers from the page. *Destruction. Devastation.* "Yes," I said.

One warm June evening, I sat in a restaurant near my home, listening intently to the sixty-something bearded man across the table.

"Now, your mother was something else in the classroom," Dr. Durand said, his Louisiana roots making two syllables of "else." "She was as like to say, 'That's the most ridiculous thing I ever heard,' when somebody proposed a proof. And then when they'd work it out on the chalkboard, you know, she'd say, 'Well, I was wrong.'"

William Durand was my mother's first EdD advisee in mathematics in the 1960s. We had met at math department picnics when he was a graduate student and I was a child. Now he was a magician, conjuring a woman I once knew.

"She was hard," he said, looking into the past above my head. "She was a *hard* teacher, but if you did your homework, you were okay." He paused. "If you didn't, well, she'd keep calling on you till you were embarrassed enough to get it done the next time. She was...*respected*. Yes, people respected her. Students. Teachers."

The clattering dishes and conversations around me disappeared as I drank in a vaguely familiar foreign language: imaginary numbers, real analysis, topology, *p*-adic integers, functions, complex variables, number theory, linear algebra. These words from my mother's vocabulary swirled in beautiful patterns in front of me, whispering of a time in the distant past, when grownups were the ones who worried and I read fairy tales.

I was not a mathematician and would never fully understand all of the words, but two glistened with new meaning: *Finite. Infinite.*

Just before we left the restaurant, Dr. Durand said, "Now, remember. Your mother touched the lives of so many people. She really made a difference."

Touching lives. I remembered seeing her hands covered in chalk dust after solving problems at the blackboard. Now she sat in a wheelchair with God-knows-what crusted brown under her fingernails.

For this gift from Dr. Durand, I forced my trembling lips into a smile. "Thank you."

My mother died from a bout of pneumonia just before midnight on May 7, 2000, a year after entering the nursing home. We had authorized an autopsy so that my mother could contribute to the knowledge base—so that she could continue to make a difference. Her brain showed changes consistent with Alzheimer's. *Probable* became *definite*.

After my mother died, I gave myself a break from learning about Alzheimer's. I wanted a *finite* experience of the disease.

But I kept learning in other areas—notably, about *love*. My mother's death brought me closer to my father. As he aged, I learned about his *chronic obstructive pulmonary disease* (COPD). He fought fungal and bacterial infections. This time, I was more prepared to be of service. I arranged to have meals delivered to his house. We spoke frankly of his will. I stayed with him often. In the last month of his life, I learned about *macrolide antibiotics* and *drug interactions*. I stood ready to move in with him, should he need it.

He didn't. And when he died, I learned that losing a parent could be simply *sad* instead of *dismal*.

5

TRANSITIONS: A CODING SECRET

from the mind of Jeanne LeCaine Agnew

Exercises are of value only to those who work them. *First, it is convenient to devise a way of setting up a message so it fits into a vector space.* Sending a message that cannot be read {except by those who know} {a coding secret} {a mundane process}: universally appealing. An object moves from a straight path *(which has an infinite radius of curvature)* to a circular path *(which has a finite radius of curvature).* The secrets of the atom are a part of this body of knowledge. Harvard was ostensibly an all-male school. This is dangerous. Many if not most natural processes remain continuous; the aging processes proceed continuously from birth to death. These integrals certainly look forbidding. {It is clear} that the integration cannot be performed in closed form. The discovery of the laws of the Universe has been our assignment since the beginning of time. *The scrambler transformation.* Mastery {of linear algebra} {*this is dangerous*} can come only by conscientiously developing problem solving {and problem posing} skills. *What is the most desirable transition curve between two straight roads of different directions in the horizontal plane?* One which provides a continuous change in the radius of curvature throughout the transition. *{A straight path} : {an infinite radius of curvature}* The reciprocal of the curvature is the radius of curvature. In general, let S be an n-dimensional linear space and let T be a linear transformation from S to S. This spot has, more than any other, been the wellspring of my life.

Source Sentences
- This spot has, more than any other, been the well-spring of my life.
- Harvard was ostensibly an all-male school.
- The discovery of the laws of the Universe has been our assignment since the beginning of time.
- The secrets of the atom are a part of this body of knowledge.

Agnew, Jeanne LeCaine. "By Choice and By Chance." *Still Running…Personal stories by Queen's women celebrating the fiftieth anniversary of the Marty Scholarship*. Joy Parr, ed. Kingston, Ontario: Queen's University Alumnae Association, 1987.

- While a great deal of attention at present centers on the role of discrete processes in the mathematics curriculum many, if not most, natural processes remain continuous.
- The aging process proceeds continuously from birth to death despite the fact that the record of aging is kept in terms of discrete numbers of years or months.
- What is the most desirable transition curve between two straight roads of different directions in the horizontal plane?
- So, according to Talbot, the most desirable transition curve is one which provides a continuous change in the radius of curvature throughout the transition.

- The reciprocal of the curvature … is called the radius of curvature.
- These integrals certainly look forbidding. It is clear that the integration cannot be performed in closed form.

Agnew, Jeanne LeCaine, and James R. Choike. "Transitions." *College Mathematics Journal* 18:2 (124–133), March 1987.

- Exercises are of value only to those who work them.
- Mastery of linear algebra can come only by conscientiously developing problem solving (and problem posing) skills.
- In general, let S be an n-dimensional linear space and let T be a linear transformation from S to S.
- Section 5.4: An Application: The Scrambler Transformation
- The idea of sending a message that cannot be read except by those who know a coding secret is universally appealing, whether one looks at the exercise as a puzzle, as part of "intelligence" and intrigue, or simply as a mundane process of transmitting restricted information.

Agnew, Jeanne LeCaine, and Robert C. Knapp. *Linear Algebra with Applications*. Belmont, CA: Wadsworth Publishing Company, 1978.

6

BACKWARDS, OPPOSITE, CONTRARY

owing: using oars to propel a boat. When you row, everything is backwards. You face away from your destination. Your right oar is to port, the boat's left side. Your left oar is to starboard, the boat's right side.

Manoeuvring feels strange at first, but with practice, your brain adjusts. As it does to so many things.

* * *

It's mid-August, and I'm visiting my parents at our family property. We're at the larger of our two camps, washing the supper dishes, when my mother starts in, her voice anxious.

"Oh-oh, it's getting late. It's ten, twenty past … past two." She compares her watch to the clock on the mantel.

My father sighs audibly.

I resist shooting him a look. He's been with her all day, I remind myself. Meanwhile, I had precious alone time all afternoon, before coming over to fix supper. I say, "Mom, it's still early. Just twenty past seven, that's all."

Her voice is doubtful. "Now, my watch says, twenty, nearly half-past seven."

I muster bright energy. "Yes, and look how much of the evening is left! Let's sit by this nice fire you've got going."

They don't need the fire—the late-summer sun still warms the room—but tending it gives Mom something to do, and its crackle adds cheer.

"Well...." Mom's dubious.

I hand her the knitting needles holding the half-finished square she's been working on. "Here—you can do this while Dad reads a chapter from our book."

Mollified but still suspicious, she plops down in her rocking chair.

"I suppose I could do a few more on this guy." She adds under her breath, "Let's see, one, two, three, then one, two," as she counts different-coloured rows. I try not to remember how intricate patterns once delighted her mathematical mind.

As Dad reads, I relax a little.

***

My father's voice always lulled me to sleep at camp. My childhood dreams were full of stories from the Old Testament, Narnia, and Middle Earth.

When we kids—my four siblings and I—grew up, we stopped reading aloud, in part because my brothers, as adults, brought their own family traditions. And although I don't have other family demands, my vacation always feels too short. I'd rather spend the evenings rowing or otherwise near the water at the smaller camp at the point, not cooped up with my parents in the larger camp around the bay.

This summer has been different, for many reasons. Mom's increased forgetfulness this spring, fifteen months after her Alzheimer's diagnosis, meant I had extra tasks, all done long- distance, to get her here. Her neurologist didn't understand why I felt so strongly about taking her to camp. I've wondered about it myself—first as I nixed my father's blithe plan to "drive up as usual" over three days from their home in Oklahoma. Instead, they flew—still a long day's travel for a couple in their early eighties—and rented a car for their stay. I wondered again as I flew to Canada from my Colorado home to open the place and fill the freezer. And I wondered yet again as I used vacation time and money I didn't have for this second trip up to support my father.

The hardest task of all has been pushing past my fears: *What if everything goes up in flames? What if a bear gets Mom and Dad? What if something else terrible happens?* I've tried to rein in my imagination to foresee and prevent actual problems.

So far, I'm glad I persevered. Mom enjoys being here.

And I'm glad to be with them, most of the time. It's hard to handle the fearful, fretful woman who replaced my brilliant, dynamic mother. My father, a short-tempered devotee of routine and predictability, has welcomed my presence, even as he's successfully adjusted to her needs in ways I couldn't have predicted. Like reading aloud in the evenings again—this year, a murder mystery by one of Mom's favourite writers.

Earlier this summer, I'd noticed that Mom didn't read for pleasure anymore. I wonder if she consciously decided to stop, frustrated by her inability to understand or remember what she read. I hope not; I hope she just put down her book one day and never thought to pick it up again.

* * *

That evening in front of the fire, I peek at Mom. She seems to feel my eyes and looks up from her work to smile. I smile back but look away quickly, so she's not tempted to interrupt.

Soon I'm drawn into the story, its plot a puzzle that can be solved.

Dad looks up at the clock without losing his place, and then flicks a glance at my mother.

She's quiet, so he moves smoothly into the next chapter.

I look toward Mom, too. From his angle, Dad can't see her trying to catch my eye. She shakes her head at me, lips drawn together. I quickly turn back to Dad. I see from the corner of my eye that Mom's knitting sits idly in her lap, and the fingers of her left hand pull at her lower lip, a sure sign of her worry. She sighs and gets up. I tense, but she only adds a log to the fire, then sits back down and picks up her knitting again.

Dad reads a little longer, then looks at the clock. It's been an hour, the upper limit of Mom's attention span. At the next stopping place, he puts in the bookmark.

"Could the daughter have done it?" I ask.

Dad thinks for a minute. "Not from what we know so far."

Mom breaks in. "We have a one here," she points to the long cot in the corner, strewn with knitted squares and yarn, "and more upstairs." She continues knitting, watching me.

I smile but raise a finger to say, "Just a sec while I finish this thought with Dad."

As I chat more with Dad, I watch Mom try to wait. She finishes out the row of knitting and then leans forward in her chair waiting for the next break in our conversation. "Because of course we have that one," and points to the cot, "and at least one other one."

My smile is polite, if a bit tight. "Yes, thank you."

She heads to the bathroom. As she comes back into the living room, she fiddles with her watch. She waits for one of us to take a breath and points at the cot. "So, would you rather this one, or I suppose you could use that one…"

I take a deep breath and say, "Thanks, Mom, but I'm not staying here tonight. I'm staying at the little camp, over at the point."

She looks at me in dismay, her black eyebrows drawn together. "Oh, no, surely not."

"Of course." I try to keep the irritation out of my voice. This is the fourth night in a row we've had this conversation, and I can answer her objections before she voices them. "It's perfectly safe. I know where everything is."

"But I just ... wouldn't you rather stay here? We have a place here, and another upstairs."

"Thanks, Mom, but no. Look, it's early yet. Wouldn't you like to sit down and talk with us?"

"Well, yes." She doesn't move. "I'd like it if you stayed here. Are you sure you want to go?"

"Yes, Mom. I love sleeping over there. I get to see you during the day."

She sighs. "Well, I suppose...." She wanders near the window before planting herself behind my chair.

I try to pick up the conversation with Dad. Mom breaks in, "You know, we have one here…"

I talk over her—rudely, firmly. "*Mom*. I'm staying at the other place."

"But I *worry* about you there."

I attempt reassurance. "I've stayed over there by myself a lot. Look, it's still very light. I'll be fine. I promise."

"Well, if you really want to, I suppose he and I could take you over, in the, the…" she points outside.

"I have my own car. See the blue one? I'll drive myself when it's time." I try to tease. "You know, I'm starting to think you want to get rid of me."

She doesn't see the joke. "No, I'm not. I want you to stay here." She checks her watch, then sighs again. She takes a couple of steps toward the cot. As her eyes fall on it, she says, "You know, we have this one…."

Dad closes his eyes and inhales deeply, then exhales.

I give up. "I guess it's time to go." I pick up my purse. Mom watches unhappily, pulling at her lower lip. I give Dad a brief hug and then go to hug her.

She reaches up to put her hands on my shoulders, and says, "Why, you're awfully tall! When did you get so tall?"

I laugh. "Twenty years ago, when I was a teenager." I kiss her cheek.

She puts her arms around me, saying, "I just *worry* about you so."

I hug her and say it yet again. "I know, Mom, but I'll be fine."

"You're sure."

I try not to shout. "Yes. Good night!"

Once down the steps, I turn to wave. They wave back, Dad's arm around Mom, comforting her. I hurry to the car. Maybe she'll stop worrying when I'm out of sight.

But I'm annoyed. Worse, her worries have stirred up the voices I've been working to keep at bay: You're not doing it right. You're not competent. You're failing.

* * *

Rowing: A sport, with defined rules and roles. A culture.

When Mom was a child and the small camp at the point was the only one, her family always had a motorboat—a wooden hull powered by a tiny engine my grandfather picked up at the dump and refreshed with spare parts. He'd taught my mother to treat the lake with respect, and she repeated his lesson to us often: "Storms can blow up giant waves out of nowhere."

When my parents were first married, my grandparents built the second camp about a kilometre away. Every summer, Mom and Dad brought their growing family to vacation at the little camp. When I was very young, my grandparents died. None of the rest of us had the skill to maintain a motorboat, so my parents didn't replace it. We had a flat-bottomed wooden rowboat for a few years, but by the time I was ten, it leaked too much to caulk, and Mom decreed its day over. After that, we had a small canoe, and although my mother allowed my then-teenaged brothers to take all-day excursions, she watched the water with what she called "a weather eye" until they were safely back home.

When I was in my mid-twenties, my parents began thinking of retirement. Mom bought a twelve-foot aluminum rowboat and fitted it with the oarlocks and oars her father had made. In the prow, she added a long heavy chain and a keyed padlock.

For this rowboat, she dictated strict rules. Unless we were out on the water, we must wrap the chain around a tree and lock the padlock. If we weren't on the beach watching, the boat must be pulled completely off the beach to keep it safe from sudden storms. The oars were to be stowed in the camp's breezeway to make it even harder for someone to steal it.

Although my siblings and I were in our twenties and thirties by this time, we rolled our eyes like teenagers, flouting some rules and obeying others only when she was around to inspect.

In spite of our wayward behaviour, we had learned the lesson. On vacation, my sister and I often stayed out in the rowboat for hours, circling islands and exploring reefs—but always keeping an eye on waves and weather.

* * *

That night after supper, back at the smaller camp, I turn on the gas light and lay a fire in the fireplace. Then I walk the few yards to the beach. The water is too choppy to take the rowboat out, so I just swat mosquitoes and watch darkness settle over the water.

When it's time for bed, I first light the fire for my own portion of cheer. As I settle into my sleeping bag, I listen to the fire crackle, its whispers as comforting as my father's voice.

* * *

The next night after supper, Mom frowns intently at her knitting while Dad reads aloud. That afternoon she'd dropped a stitch, and fixing it has required her full concentration. She's been focused and absorbed all evening.

At the end of the chapter, I say to Dad, "Well, now it sounds like the son did it."

Dad shakes his head. "He couldn't have been the mugger, and that's what led to the murder."

"Hmm, you're right." I glance at Mom. "How's the knitting coming?"

"Oh, fine." She holds it up to show me, pointing to an uneven spot. "This doesn't look too good, but I guess it will do."

I lean forward to pick up the end. "You did a good job of fixing it. If you don't say anything, nobody will notice." Kind if not true.

"Well, it's not too, too much or anything, but I enjoy it. Say, it's nearly, nine. Nine o'clock? Can that be right?"

I look up. "Yes, it is. I'd better get home."

"You're going home?" Mom is surprised.

"Well, to the other place, at the point. I'm staying there this week."

"Oh, you are." Her busy fingers finish her row. "And you're not scared to stay alone?"

I smile. "Not at all. I know where everything is there, and I feel very safe."

She sighs. "Well, if you're sure…."

"I am, Mom." I gather my purse and jacket.

Mom puts down her knitting and gets up to say goodnight. As I hug her, she says, "Would you like us…we could go in the…."

She seems so tiny. "Thanks, Mom, but I have my own car. See you tomorrow!"

I hug and kiss Dad. As I drive away, they wave from the window. I say aloud, "So much more pleasant! See how unnecessary all that worry is?"

But back at the point, I feel restless. I rinse my coffee mug and take out the garbage. I pick up my book and put it down. Finally, I head outdoors to collect sticks for the fireplace. The sunset behind the camp trails reddish-orange fire across the water to an island in the bay.

In just a few minutes, I'm rowing through the majestic evening, following the sunset's path. Automatically adjusting my stroke for the greater strength in my right arm, I skim across the water, trying to outdistance my agitation and unhappiness.

The big lake is nearly calm. Even when the sun itself disappears beyond the trees, the evening sky dazzles my eyes and turns the water around me an opaque platinum. A breeze ruffles the water's surface, shooting lilac and iridescent highlights along the tops of the ripples.

With each stroke, my dripping oars create new patterns of pink-rimmed circles that grow, overlap, and fade.

Time slows. So does my pace. So does my anxious heart.

Finally, I rest my oars and sit quietly. A slight swell moves the water beneath me. I inhale and exhale, matching the lake's breath.

* * *

Rowing: A pastime. An activity. A way to get from here to there. Except you can't see where you're going. Only where you've been.

When my parents finally retired completely, they stayed at the bigger place my grandparents had built around the curve of the bay, out of sight of the small camp. Mom's disease has transformed her respect for the lake into fear. Earlier this summer, I took her out for a row once or twice, but she fretted and complained. Another loss, like her lost pleasure in mathematical patterns and in reading, but somehow deeper and more painful for the rest of us.

* * *

Ripples murmur against the rowboat's hull as the lake and I breathe together. The sky darkens. I look over my shoulder at the island's black silhouette. It's time to turn around. As I row in, I watch new stars pierce the indigo sky.

I'm no longer restless, but sadness still lies along my shoulders, feather-light but impossible to ignore.

Back at the beach, I pull the boat up, far beyond the recent high-water mark, though not as far as Mom would demand. I wrap the boat's chain around a tree, ignoring the padlock. She'd be furious if she knew I haven't used the lock in several years. I lean the oars against the house, feeling momentary guilt at not bringing them into the breezeway.

Indoors, I light the usual fire and zip myself into my sleeping bag, but I'm not sleepy. Instead, I watch the sky through the bank of windows and wait for the moon to rise. I can still feel the movement of the boat in my bones.

The thought surfaces: *She sure worries about that boat.* And then it clicks.

She wasn't as worried about me tonight. That's what felt wrong—backwards, opposite, contrary. When she worries about me, I feel insulted. But when she doesn't worry, I feel bereft—as if she doesn't care.

As the fire crackles away, I mull over Mom's illness, our worries, our desire to keep each other safe. As always, I wish I could heal her. But maybe navigating these waters with her is enough. In any case, it's all I know to do.

7

HOURS OF DAYLIGHT (I)

This is the story of my mother's first day of school.
It's January of 1924, halfway between my mother's sixth and seventh birthdays. My grandmother has been teaching both my mother and my uncle at their home in Port Arthur, Ontario. She thinks Mom is ready for Grade 2, but the Grade 1 teacher requires convincing.

The teacher says to Mom, "The earth is round like an orange, slightly flattened at both ends. Can you say that back to me?"

My mother replies, "The earth is an oblate spheroid."

She is put into Grade 2. By the end of that year, she is in Grade 3 with her older brother.

* * *

This is a story of nights that are broken in hard-to-understand ways.

More than seventy years later, in the family home in Oklahoma, I'm sound asleep when footsteps and the creak of hardwood floors pull me toward wakefulness. I recognize the special squeak of the door to the hallway bathroom, near my parents' bedroom across the landing. Water murmurs.

But I'm far away and drifting farther, drowsing.

Then I hear Dad's voice saying something like "What?" and suddenly I'm alert. I hold my watch in the orange shaft of light slanting in from the streetlight. It's 2:15. I struggle to orient myself. Right. I'm at my parents' home, visiting.

Mom must be up. Why is she in the hallway bathroom instead of the small bathroom off the master bedroom? Yes, the hallway bathroom has a tub, and she prefers baths to showers, but it's the middle of the night. She can't be taking a bath…can she?

Dad's voice is loud but I can't distinguish his words through my closed bedroom door. Should I get up? To do what, exactly? I shiver.

The bathroom door opens, and now Dad's words are bullet-hard. "Come on. No, you are going *back* to *bed*."

Mom's voice, muffled, rises in pitch.

Dad answers, "No. It's night. Come. To. Bed."

Mom murmurs and I hear water draining. Then shuffling—Mom's slippered feet on the hardwood of the hallway—and Dad's even, measured steps. Silence when they enter their carpeted bedroom.

I lie back down, eyes wide. I should have expected this. I've read about it—sundowning, the agitation and sleep problems common at Mom's stage of Alzheimer's. I just didn't think it would be like this, though I don't know what I'd envisioned. I feel as if I'm always off-kilter. I can't imagine how it feels to Mom.

Earlier that day, we'd met with my parents' lawyer to assign powers of attorney. I knew, and I suspect their attorney also knew, that Mom didn't understand what she signed, but none of us acknowledged it. There wasn't anything to say.

Mom had always been so sure of herself, an instigator of structure, rules, and schedules. Although she complained of feeling awkward at parties, she enjoyed hosting meetings related to mathematics and teaching, her great loves. Around our dining room table, she gathered her younger math department colleagues to brainstorm ideas for grants. Each semester, she hosted a dinner at which her undergraduate applied math students met with mathematicians who had jobs in industries outside academe, where they solved real-world problems.

And Mom made peace with social expectations. Every December, the United Methodist Women's Christmas party was at our house. The dining room table, fully extended, was also fully loaded. A punchbowl stood at one end, a silver tea and coffee service at the other, and the surface between was paved with homemade sweets—mint brownies, toffee, chocolate-covered cherries, divinity, fudge, orange/coconut cookies, candy-cane cookies, spiced and sugared pecans.

But during my March visit, the days of Mom's teaching and hostessing are years in the past. Paper has sifted into the house, and now the dining room table is piled with mail and magazines and catalogues and programs and church bulletins. Dad gives me a protracted sidelong glance when I move a few stacks to make room for my place at mealtime.

I'm the youngest of their five children, and only the three of us—Mom, Dad, and me—were home together during my high school years. As a teenager, I was sullen, more withdrawn than overtly rebellious. After I went away to college, I became again their obedient daughter. A period of soul-searching in my late twenties worried them, but when I finished graduate school and found work I enjoyed 800 miles away, we became comfortable together again.

Still, in this house where I grew up, whose every shift and groan is familiar to me, where my swimming trophies and music awards perch on the shelves, I can't find my thirty-seven-year-old adult self. In the face of Mom's illness, I'm afraid. As my vibrant mother disappears, I struggle to find a way to help her. What can I do? What if I only make her disease worse?

And how do I support my father? He's a bookish historian and usually a gentle man, but he's always had a temper. When we were young, he was impatient and cranky when asked to alter his routines. But he and Mom never fought—in fact, they never disagreed in front of us. So, led by Mom, we all adjusted to him.

When Mom's illness first appeared, she repeated stories and lost words. Now she's also agitated and afraid in the late afternoon, and she wakes up at night. Understandably, Dad's showing the strain of caring for her. I've seen him angry more often during this visit than I ever have before.

"Helping Mom and Dad" feels possible in the abstract, until I'm actually with them.

* * *

This is the story of lengthening days.

March includes the equinox, the balancing point when day and night are the same length. In Oklahoma that year, March 16th has eleven hours and fifty-nine minutes of daylight; March 17th has twelve hours and two minutes.

Day by day, the amount of daylight changes only gradually. Nevertheless, these changes accumulate. Eventually, minutes become hours.

On that visit to my parents, crocuses and hyacinths have awakened from winter and pushed through the soil to bloom. Jonquils and the forsythia bush are budding.

It feels particularly cruel to watch my mother's life diminish during the spring, when everything around us speaks to a promise of new life. When everything she is to me, everything and everyone she ever has been—they're all slipping through my fingers.

I think, too, of all the versions of me that she'll never live to see.

* * *

This is a story of unmet expectations.

In the bedroom I used to share with my sister, I find a manila file folder labelled "Hours of Daylight." The words, pencilled in my mother's strong handwriting, are from a previous era. The folder, now empty, once held notes for one of the applied mathematics problems she and her colleagues collected.

But I don't know what the mathematics problem actually was—which company in which industry it came from, what they needed to know and why, what level of mathematics the students used to define and solve the problem. I don't remember asking. My parents' lives were so often simply wallpaper to mine.

Perhaps, out of politeness, I did ask, and Mom told me. I didn't retain it. She wanted me to be a mathematician—as her youngest child, I was her last hope, she used to say—but she also thought the elegance of mathematics, its different language that gives a different perspective on the world, would enthrall me the way it had her.

But like my historian father, I'm a dreamer and reader. I liked mathematics fine, but I didn't inherit my mother's tenacity, her ability to work at a knotty problem past the point of exhaustion to arrive at understanding. I never imagined a career in mathematics—only in some field that let me read and write.

* * *

This is a story of fury and furies.

The next night, Mom gets up three times to go the hallway bathroom. Each time I hear her, I hold my breath until she shuffles back to the master bedroom. I wonder whether Dad wakes up, too.

At breakfast, we sit bleary-eyed over the standard morning meal—cereal, toast, and coffee, followed by a devotional reading. My father and I are never cheerful in the morning, and my mother, who once loved mornings, seems unusually subdued. I decide to take Mom for a walk this afternoon, after church and lunch. Maybe that will help us all get some sleep.

Mom pushes her chair back from the table and stands up. She smooths her skirt and heads toward the stairs.

"Here, where are you going?" Dad snaps. "We haven't read the *Upper Room* yet. Get back here."

I cringe in my chair, croaking out, "Hey."

He yells over me. "Get over here and sit down."

In one motion, he pushes his chair back and is at Mom's side. I half-stand. He places his hands lightly on her shoulders and steers her back to her chair.

Mom and I sit down at the same time. She stares at her plate, her mouth drawn, and picks up her knife to sweep toast crumbs into small piles.

Meanwhile, Dad marks the devotion booklet with a ballpoint pen from the stash in his shirt pocket. Then he reads aloud.

Tension buzzes in my ears, drowning out his words. I flinch when he thrusts the book at Mom.

"Here." His voice is sharp. He points to the spot where she should begin reading.

She reads without inflection, stumbling over "appreciate" and "Thessalonians." She doesn't seem to understand what she reads, but she's far more fluent reading than speaking.

She hands the book to me. I say "Prayer," and "Amen," and "Thought for the Day," and in between, a host of other words I hardly hear. When I reach the bottom of the page, I close the booklet and hand it across the table to Dad.

Mom stands up again. This time, I go upstairs with her. At the top, I say softly, "Mom, can I ask you something?"

She pauses in the doorway of the master bedroom. "Yes, sure."

I swallow but say it. "When Dad yells at you like that, do you mind?"

She half-laughs and says, "Oh, I don't ... so, so tott."

I rest a hand on her shoulder so she'll look me in the face. "Really, Mom. Does it upset you?"

She sighs. "Not so much. He's stotting things, you know, and he, he wants me to—well—sarft something, in a good way. He does a good job."

"Well, if you get upset, let me know, okay?"

"Okay." She smiles and the pucker in her forehead smooths. I rejoice, silently, to see her relax.

But my glow fades as I dress for church. Even if she understood what I was talking about in that moment, she won't remember when she gets upset.

Still, I said something. I tried to help.

That Sunday afternoon, my walk with Mom starts slowly. On our sidewalk, she stops to lament the overgrown front garden. If I'm going to tire her out, we need to meander less and walk more.

"Okay, Mom, let's go!" I slip my hand through her arm. She smiles at me, and as we walk, I can't help but cheer up. The sunny day feels more like May than March. Remarking on the neighbours' gardens, we follow the street around the curve and downhill, then turn right. At the stoplight, we could turn uphill toward home or continue for another short block before taking a different street up to the house. Without asking, I decide we're going on.

"But, no," Mom says. "We want to go here." She walks in front of me so I'll turn.

"We're just starting. How about we go another block." I still have her arm, so I gently lead her across the street.

Once across, she tries to turn up the hill again.

I try to sound patient. "Mom, this way. Come on." She pulls away from me, and I grab her hand.

"Oh, all right." She walks with me. "But Mother won't like it."

Mother? But…*Grandma died thirty years ago.* Cold with fear, I look at her. "You mean Dad?" I hesitate to refer to my father by his first name. "Ted?"

"No, *Mother*." She shakes her head, impatient. "She'll wonder where we are."

"Well, *Dad* knows we're on a walk."

She says, slowly and distinctly, "Mother. Doesn't."

We continue walking. That is, I walk, and I have her arm, so she comes along.

As we pass another garden, she moans, "Oh, Mother won't *like* this. We need to *go home.*"

I turn to face her, my words cruel. "Mom, your mother is dead." I take a breath and go on. "*Dad,* your husband, *Ted,* knows we're on a walk. It's okay." I walk on, still holding her arm.

Beside me, her voice is small but defiant. "No. It's not okay. Mother will be angry."

At the next corner, she says, "Here, now. This way." She turns toward home, yanking her arm from my grasp, her step purposeful—I can't tell what force is pulling her up the hill, but it's powerful. I have to speed up.

We face the afternoon sun, still high in the sky. A sadness rises in my chest. I had thought that my presence, if nothing else, would be of some comfort my mother. But I don't know how or where she feels at home and safe—or, selfishly, where I do, either.

When we're within sight of our driveway, she stops again to point out another garden. Whatever internal Fate or Fury that has driven her to "go home to Mother" has fallen silent. Once again, she speaks pleasantly, if vaguely, about blooms and stems and leaves.

* * *

This is a story of losing stories.

My mother has written two university-level mathematics textbooks. She's written at least a dozen sets of curricula for applied mathematics problems for university students, many research papers about neutron transport equations, and a biographical essay for an anthology celebrating a women's scholarship at Queen's University, where she earned her B.A. and M.A. in Mathematics.

She wrote family stories of her childhood and youth in Port Arthur, Ontario, in the years between the World Wars. She collated these stories, searching out and copying old family photographs, and gave them to my siblings and me.

But I can't find any publication or manuscript where she wrote the story of her first day at school.

We know it, of course. The family—my father, my siblings and I, and other people she knows well—we all know that story. It has been left to me to write it down.

* * *

This is a story of hopes and horrors.

The night after our walk, the sound of running water wakes me. *So much for the walk helping her sleep.*

Pulling on sweatpants and sweatshirt, I creep to my half-open bedroom door. The light is on at the top of the stairs. I hide behind my door, listening to Dad's raised voice.

"Now. This instant. You are *com*ing to *bed*."

"Get out of here." My mother's voice is low and rough, a bear's growl. I gasp. I've never heard her like this, not even when I misbehaved as a child. I've certainly never heard her speak this way to my father.

Dad sounds like he's strangling. "You will—get—come here." I hear scuffling. At the same time, Mom's bear-voice says, "It's terrible, it's awful."

I burst onto the landing. Near the door to the girls' bathroom, Dad stands behind Mom, again holding both of her upper arms. She twists, trying to free herself from his grasp.

I say, shakily, "Hey, what's the matter?"

Mom sees me and quits struggling. She is near tears. "He—I was—and then he—comes *right* in, and it's, it's not, not *right*."

Dad's voice is loud but calm. "Come to bed." He drops his hands from her arms and holds out a hand. "Come on." She doesn't move, so he picks up her hand from her side and leads her into the bedroom. She follows him without protest.

I stand on the landing, looking after them. The light in their bedroom is off, and the landing light shines only a few feet into the room.

I can't go in. Whatever my age, or theirs, they're my parents, and I can't intrude.

I turn off the landing light.

Back in my room, I crawl into bed, sweats and all. I curl up in a ball, still shivering, then check my watch: 3:30. Not that it matters. Mom doesn't even know what year it is. She doesn't recognize her husband. She wouldn't believe I'm her child.

I shut my eyes against the beam from the street light. Exhausted, I drift off.

Just a few hours after Mom's harsh-voiced encounter with Dad, we're meeting with a neuropsychologist, Dr. Whatley.

Mom's neurologist suggested individual neuropsychological appointments for both Mom and Dad, but Dad hasn't made an appointment for himself. As he explained to me on the phone a few weeks earlier, Dr. Whatley is "only" a Ph.D., not an M.D., so he couldn't offer Dad any *medical* advice.

I kept my eye-roll out of my voice. "Maybe he could give you advice about coping."

"Mmmm," Dad had said. Meaning *Hmph*.

Mom has disappeared with a nurse while Dad and I sit in the waiting room. I'm frustrated. We'll never know what Dr. Whatley is saying to her. Mom can't carry a message or describe what happened. I should have gone with her. I should have insisted.

Misery balls in my stomach as I brood. I still haven't done anything concrete to help my parents, and I'm flying home immediately after this appointment.

Next to me, Dad mutters, "Was that Wednesday? Yes, I think it was." He's filling out a form on a clipboard. He adds, "Before last night, the last time she had one of those episodes of, what's-it-called, sundowning, was last week."

"How about Friday? And on Saturday night, she was up a lot."

"She did go back to bed, both nights."

I try not to stare at him. "She was up three times. And Friday, she ran bath water." The fact that he talked her out of getting into the tub is a technicality. He can't play fast and loose with the truth.

"Oh, all right," he says, as if I am being completely unreasonable.

I feel my irritation rising in response to his. I stay silent and breathe.

"But the last time she *stayed* up was before you came, which would make it, let's see, Wednesday night." He heaves a sigh. "You know, my memory isn't what it used to be."

His memory? Sweet Jesus, I could kill him. In the neurologist's office where his brilliant wife is being treated for her Alzheimer's disease, *he* complains about *his* memory?

At that moment, I hate him as I never have before, not even when I was a sulky teenager. Then, the very fact of his existence—his index cards, his different colours of ballpoint pens, his routines, the fact that he and Mom were the age of my friends' grandparents—made my life a nightmare of adolescent, immature embarrassment. Even so, never has he been as loathsome to me as he is at this moment.

I bite my lips to keep from voicing the poison I feel. I fan my hot face with a magazine. While I seethe, Dad happily mutters his way through the rest of the form.

Inhale, exhale. At least he didn't complain about his memory in front of Mom; that's all I can find to be grateful for.

* * *

This is a story of holding on to grace as night falls.

Sunset doesn't create instant darkness. It creates twilight, a grace period. After sunset, the upper atmosphere still provides light—enough light to do some things, but not others.

Twilight is divided into three phases. In civil twilight, you can still see objects clearly, without artificial light. During nautical twilight, the horizon is visible even on moonless nights, and mariners navigate by the stars. Throughout astronomical twilight, the last phase, the sun's scattered light fades until it's less visible than starlight.

That March, I try to calculate where the sun is in the immense sky that has been Mom's intellect, her spirit, her life. Can she still see the horizon? Does she even look? I wonder whether waking at night frightens her. I hope the stars give her enough light that she can find some form of comfort.

Her handwriting on a file folder label, in a notebook, on an envelope (especially on an envelope, where she's written my name, firm and clear)—when I find these scraps of who she once was, I grasp them tightly.

* * *

This is a story of listening, of speaking.

Dr. Whatley finally calls us back to his inner office. He sits on a rolling stool and motions us into chairs lined up against the wall. I settle between my parents.

He says, "I've been collecting data on Mrs. Agnew for a report I'll put in her file."

I try not to wince; Mom was always known as "Dr. Agnew" until her illness. It seems pointless to bring it up.

He looks at me. "Do you live here in town?"

I feel guilty. "No, I'm just visiting." I clear my throat. "I do try to come regularly."

"Ah," he says, turning to Dad. "Then I'll need to see you to follow up on some things. Did you fill out—oh, good." Dad hands him the clipboard. He sets it aside. "I'll read that over later. I may have some follow-up questions when you come in."

Mom says, as if she's reminding Dr. Whatley of something, "And tott's a ... serf one, too."

He turns toward her and looks her in the eye. In spite of calling her "Mrs.," he's the only physician who seems to see a person—if not the gifted professor and mathematician, perhaps still the teacher who brooked no nonsense and accepted nothing sloppy, or the parent who never passed up an opportunity to urge us to harder work and greater ambition.

He answers her, "Yes, that's right."

To Dad and me, he adds, "I'm afraid I wore her out earlier. I was asking questions and she let me know she was done answering. She has very definite opinions to share, don't you?" He shoots her a smile.

She chuckles. "Yes, I spot ... spatt so."

He turns back to us, with an air of dusting his hands. "So, that's it for this time. Do you have questions?"

Dad shakes his head. I look at Dr. Whatley, debating. *I like how he is with Mom. But can I talk to him about Dad?*

We get up, and I fall back to let Mom and Dad leave before me.

I have to. I turn to the doctor. "Could I just—for a second—ask—"

"Sure," he says. "Come sit down."

We sit and I take a breath. "When you see Dad, could you talk about...." Tears fill my voice. I say, indistinctly, "Anger." Then words rush out. "She's sundowning more than he admits. And he's angry all the time, just *all* the *time*. She tries not to get upset. Lord knows I can't blame Dad, she repeats everything and gets anxious and annoying, but still, he yells and then she feels so bad."

I stop for breath and will myself into coherence. "I'm sorry; it's just hard to…to be here."

Dr. Whatley rocks a little on his stool. "I understand. It's tough."

I gulp, betrayal and fear bitter in my mouth, but I go on. "It's like he's blaming her. But she's not trying to annoy him. She's *sick*. He doesn't seem to *get* that." The tears spill out of my eyes again. I blink and take the tissue he hands me. I blow my nose.

"Thank you for letting me know," Dr. Whatley says. "I'll talk about coping mechanisms at his appointment. Is he getting any support?"

"Like what?" After the tears, I can hardly think. Everything feels hopeless.

"Like caregiver support meetings, or taking your mother to the new adult day centre."

"Oh. He's mentioned them, but he hasn't done anything."

"The day centre is really important. She'll get stimulation and one-on-one attention, and he'll get a break from dealing with her all the time."

I nod. "You'll have to be the one to tell him, though. Even if I say it, he won't hear it from me." *And maybe not from you either*, I don't add. I pull myself together and thank him.

Back in the lobby, I pass Dad, who's standing at the desk.

"Making your own appointment with Dr. Whatley?" I say loudly, hoping the receptionist will take my hint.

Mom sits in a chair in the waiting area, knees together, hands folded on top of her handbag in her lap. She stares down at her hands, her lower lip trembling.

I sit down beside her and rub her back. "How are you doing, Mom?" I wipe my cheek with the wadded up tissue I'm still holding.

"So-so," she says. Her voice is sad and small.

"Yeah." I put my arm around her. "Me too."

She speaks so softly I almost miss it. "They think I'm in a bad way."

I don't know what to say—it would feel disrespectful to contradict the truth—so I rub her back, murmuring, "It's okay, you're okay," while wishing it were true.

* * *

This is a story of resignation.

Later that afternoon, as I drive to the airport, fighting drowsiness, I admit that Mom and Dad may not have been the only ones affected by interrupted sleep and worry. I too might have become crabby and unreasonable that weekend.

But I haven't exaggerated Mom's illness, nor Dad's irritated response—his fatigue, his temper.

Although the hours of daylight in Oklahoma will continue to increase until late in June, Mom will never regain any of the abilities she's losing. Her sundowning phase is followed by more declines and more loss, my father's heart breaking a little every day as she fades away.

This is a story of unexpected connections in the dark.

For what turned out to be the last of her eighty-three years, my mother moved into Grace Living Center, a nursing home. Although Mom could still walk, she had stopped taking initiative and seemed content to sit in a wheelchair.

Her fingers remained restless, as if she'd like to turn the pages of one of her mysteries. But by this point in her disease, she was unable to read, beyond sounding out words that she no longer understood: *Galatians, accommodate.*

We looked for ways to keep Mom busy, ways to stay connected to her. My sister bought an aluminum jelly roll pan and some plastic letters and numbers, with magnets on the back. Mom enjoyed fiddling with them. During her year at Grace, she often lined them up into precisely marching rows of gibberish: TE1JKSLIRS. 2G5HR3EA.

One yellow-hot July afternoon, I perched on the edge of her bed as she sat in her wheelchair. Idly, I picked up the tray and spelled JEANNE, moving the extra letters and numbers out to the edges of the tray so that her name sat alone and grand in the centre.

"Hey, Mom," I said.

She sat in a blue cotton housedress, her feet in slippers, her glasses long gone. She rested her chin in one hand and stared toward the open door of her room.

"Mom?"

Surely she could hear me—she was close enough—but she didn't react to my voice. I reached to touch her solid forearm, saying "Mom?" She turned her head toward me, her face blank. "What's this?" I held the tray in her line of vision.

She took in a quick breath before smiling at me, her blue eyes snapping with delight.

"Why, that's *Zehn*," she said, giving her name the French pronunciation her mother had used when Mom was growing up.

She reached for the tray and grasped it. "That's me."

In the stifling heat of the room, I went cold. She was Mom no longer. She didn't recognize the name that my siblings and I had called her for nearly fifty years. Yet she was still Jeanne, her mother's daughter.

She gazed at the colourful circus of plastic letters and poked at the last E with her knobby forefinger. Still staring at the tray, she frowned briefly, and then her face relaxed into an impassive mask. Slowly, she turned her head back toward the doorway. The tray sagged into her lap. I took it from her hands before it drifted to the floor.

I sat and fingered the letters and blinked back my tears. With a sigh, I set the tray on the table beside her bed.

From that point on, I was never sure she knew my name or that I was her daughter. I didn't ask or test her, to preserve my dignity as much as her own.

Still, when she saw me, she showed pleasure, as if she knew somehow that I mattered to her—that I belonged to her, or perhaps she to me. Of course that tenuous connection wasn't really enough, but it was what I had, and I held on to it.

8

THE TENNESSEE WALTZ

I pause in front of the door to take one last breath of the damp, warm Oklahoma morning. Its sweetness will dissipate as the sun climbs the sky. I'm ready to enter. I pull the door open.

ACT I

I welcome the cooled air in the nursing home lobby on my bare legs. The smell is more difficult to accept: the sharp bite of human waste and perspiration under aggressive floral deodorizer.

I wonder if I'd still notice the smell if I visited every day—if I lived here, in the same town as my parents. The hometown I couldn't wait to leave, the hometown I never wanted to return to, a place I escaped by moving three states away. The hometown where I never felt I fit in, where I more easily understood characters in books set in England or New England than my own neighbours. Where my family still, always, seemed slightly "other," even though my parents had lived there for fifty years.

You can't think about that, I tell myself for the millionth time. *Your home and responsibilities are elsewhere. All you can do is make the most of these visits.*

I pass residents in wheelchairs and remember to smile.

One of the women holds up her arms as I pass. "Honey, I just love that dress. Those white spots on the red—it's so bright and cheerful!"

I bend to take both her hands in mine and allow my voice to slow into a drawl to match hers. "Well, thank you, ma'am. I thought it would be just right for the July Fourth weekend." I actually love the dress, too—lightweight knit, short sleeves, twirly skirt, meant for moving in. I feel almost carefree, like a little girl.

Her smile reflects in her eyes. "Your dad's here, in the dining room with your mother."

We squeeze hands and let go.

Although I'm surprised she recognizes me—we met only briefly, just the evening before—I'm glad someone here watches out for my parents.

"Thank you," I say again.

And, scene.

I find my parents and bend to kiss Mom's cheek before settling into a wooden dining chair next to the wheelchair, her "new normal" since her seizures. She can walk, but usually doesn't, and never asks to.

I make sure I speak to her. "How was your breakfast?"

Dad answers. "She ate all the oatmeal. She's just finishing her juice." He holds the glass to Mom's mouth. She takes a swallow. Her hands are closed around her "seat belt," the restraining strap that keeps her in her wheelchair, but she's not fidgeting with it at the moment. Her clear blue eyes look straight ahead of her, not at Dad or me.

He asks, "You found everything all right?"

"Yes, thanks." He left our family home by 7:00, in time to feed Mom breakfast. I followed at a more leisurely pace. I add, "I even found a coffee shop with good espresso."

He grins and shakes his head. "You'd have never made it in the Navy. That coffee would eat the bowl of your spoon right off."

Ah, yes. His Navy days. "You're right, and not just because of the coffee. I remember what you said about Navy showers. I like my coffee sweet and my showers luxurious, even on hot days."

Mom hears the teasing in my voice and turns her head toward me to smile. I swear she gives me the ghost of a wink, but I'm probably imagining it. I'm glad Dad and I know our lines—it seems to please her.

Dad gives her another sip. "Did I see Mrs. Williams stop you on your way in?"

"The lady who sat behind us last night?"

"Yes, she's one of the, ah, more capable residents here. She's lived here two years, she told me. Claims to like it." We're starting Mom's second month, still adjusting to the routines, trying to learn who her new neighbours are in this community-within-their-town.

"That's always good to hear," I offer. A pleasantry, a platitude, a thing one says.

"Uh-huh," Mom says. Momentarily surprised, I look to see if she's actually following the conversation, but she's gazing toward the kitchen. It seems to have been a random comment.

ACT II

The hair on the side of Mom's head is smashed flat, and the front is drooping toward her eyes. *Something I can fix!* "What say I brush your hair a little?"

As I speak, I hear even more Oklahoma in my voice—the vowels lengthen and idioms creep in. I never spoke like my school friends when I lived here, but now that I live elsewhere, I seem unable to rid myself of these markers completely. Well, never mind; no better place for it.

I stand, but before I can unlock Mom's wheelchair, Dad says, "Can you do it here? The calendar says they're having special music in twenty minutes, and it doesn't seem worth taking her to her room. She's comfortable here."

"Sure." I head off to collect Mom's hairbrush.

As I enter her room, her roommate, Ermal, greets me from her bed: "Guess what she did last night?"

"No telling." My voice invites the story, making the words the equivalent of "Do tell!" in other parts of the country.

Ermal is recuperating from a stroke, which has left her left side paralyzed and muffled her speech a little. Her mind, though, is clear, which makes her the perfect roommate for Mom, though they never knew each other before now. Never did, and never would have, though they crossed paths. Mom was a professor of mathematics at Oklahoma State University; Ermal worked at the cafeteria in the OSU Student Union, eventually becoming its manager.

Now she motions across the hall with her good hand, showing me Mom's escapade from the night before.

"She got up an' went over there." Her short white hair billows around her face. "I's sleepin', but somebody cried out an' woke me. It was the man in that bed. Scared him. I saw her bed's empty an' hit the call button but they didn't come, so I's blowing my kazoo, and they come runnin'. They brought her back. And then she lay down an' slep lak a baby. But I's awake for hours."

I bite my lips together. Although Ermal's stories seem meant to be entertaining, they usually involve Mom disrupting Ermal's sleep. I hide a smile and offer more pleasantries. "Sorry she woke you up. It's a good thing you had your kazoo."

Ermal waves off my apology with a short laugh. "Don't matter. I can sleep today." She motions toward Mom's empty bed. "I know she wouldn't be doin' these things if she was in her right mind."

Ouch. I re-paste my smile into place. "Yes, and thanks for watching out for her. Well, I'll let you sleep." I escape.

Ermal's right, of course. Mom's not in her right mind. We all know it. Sometimes I need to think of something else, to look for positive things. Mom ate a good breakfast. There will be special music.

Back in the dining room, I brush Mom's hair and spray it with the hairspray I had brought that morning. We've arranged for her to have her hair washed and set once a week, but it needs more attention than it gets. I debate leaving hairspray in her room. Dad visits every day, sometimes twice a day, but would he use it? Would anyone on the staff have time?

While I'm working with brush and spray, Dad takes Mom's bib and her breakfast tray into the kitchen.

I straighten the collar on Mom's blouse. The aides dressed her up some today, for the holiday. She's in a blouse and skirt instead of one of those shapeless, snap-front dusters we got for her, the kind of housedress other mothers might wear but she never did. Till now.

Dad returns from the kitchen. "Much better."

Mom lifts her head at exactly the right moment as he leans in, and their lips meet in a brief kiss. I wonder if it's a reflex, built on how many millions of kisses like that they've shared. Every time we sat down to a meal, every time one of them left the house—a public, ceremonial kiss. I turn my thoughts away from their private kisses, now past.

ACT III

The three of us watch a few men in white dress shirts and dark dress slacks set up an electronic keyboard and some microphones at one end of the room. They connect amplifiers and run cords.

I keep wondering what to say to Mom. Her fingers pull gently on her lower lip, a habit that once meant she was worried or deep in thought, but she doesn't look anxious. Maybe she doesn't know she does it anymore.

It feels odd to not know how to connect with her. Long before her illness, our relationship had become comfortable, far more comfortable than in the days when she nagged me to aspire higher and work harder. As adults, we could talk about many things—not quite anything or everything, but close.

Dad, always, has been more difficult. Difficult to talk to. Difficult to connect with—off in the study, lost in a book, frowning at a clipboard while scratching notes in ballpoint pen. When we did interact, he leaned heavily on the *acting* part, always just a little *too* hearty, disappointed, or happy, his grin a little *too* wide, his frown and head-shake a little *too* emphatic.

After I left home, the phone lines kept us in touch. "Hi, Daddy, how are you?"

"Oh, fine." We might exchange a weather report. And then after a moment, he'd either say, "I'll get your mother" or I'd ask if she was there, and that would be that. Regular, but brief.

Even in person, he and I conversed best when Mom was there, too, and not yet sick. We'd linger over a meal at the dining room table, telling each other our family's stories, going back a century or two, sometimes circling back to the present. News about family—say, sibling fights among my nieces and nephews—sometimes prompted new-to-me stories from his own childhood, his three brothers and two sisters, all younger, and the pressure of being the oldest, the example representing the family, the forced lessons in violin and elocution.

I grew to understand that he loved me, though I didn't always feel it. And of course we never spoke of it. My friends' fathers, in shorts and tennis shoes and golf shirts, slung their arms around my friends' shoulders for a squeeze and a hearty-voiced, "Love ya, punkin," but we—well, we didn't. Any of that.

And then Mom's dementia became impossible to ignore and impossible to fix. Dad and I clashed about the best way to care for her, which was presumptuous on my part, given that he was the one doing the work. His impatience with Mom upset her and me, and probably him as well. Our disagreements also seemed to make Mom's agitation worse.

As Mom's dementia grew, Dad and I made an effort to speak civilly to each other, but we grew icy. Just a few weeks ago, when he acquiesced to nursing-home care for her, the silences between us thawed slightly. A beginning—the start of what must become new patterns, someday, when we no longer have Mom at all. Which neither of us wants to imagine.

And we both still have tender spots. So we speak with care, relying on the safe things to say, older stories, affectionate banter, and gentle respect.

Mom seems to feel more relaxed, too, although it's hard to know.

The music begins, quieting the buzz of chatter in the room. One man plays the keyboard while another sings. A third man sits behind the speakers, sullen, frowning at his feet. His manner irritates me, so I focus on the others.

The singer is about sixty, with a pleasant, pink face and a fringe of white hair around his bald spot. He croons a medley of gospel songs. They sound vaguely familiar, but not enough for Dad or me to sing along. When he's done, we and the other visitors lead the applause, while a few of the residents join in.

Mom claps, too, suddenly, a little late, her dark eyebrows drawn together in concentration.

I lean over to her, and she stops. "He sounded good, didn't he?"

Mom says, "Star tuff and some, I don't know," and chuckles.

I pat her arm. It's what I do.

He plays the chorus of "In My Merry Oldsmobile," making eye contact with the front row, then sings a verse. Several of the residents keep time, patting the tables or the arms of their wheelchairs. He finishes to more applause—warm and real.

I glance at Mom. She's still looking at her hands and doesn't clap.

ACT IV

The balding man strums a little to ease into the next song.

"Now then, time for a little dancing. I'm going sing about my favourite place, my home state of Tennessee, 'The Tennessee

Waltz,' and I want y'all to just get on up and dance if you feel like it."

They start the waltz. Dad says, across Mom, "Hey, we should be dancing. Come on." He gets up and holds out a hand to me.

"I don't know how." I stand anyway.

"I'll do my best to show you."

"Okay, but I don't follow well." Probably not something I need to say. Especially to him.

We find an open spot near the musicians. At Dad's direction, I hold up my right hand and put my left on his shoulder. We're the same height. He was never tall—five-ten at most. Now, at eighty-two, he's the five-seven he claims only when he stands straight.

"*One*-two-three, *one*-two-three," he says. "Step out on *one*. Like a box."

He and I have never danced together, not like other little girls in fancy dresses, standing on their daddy's feet. Not to practise before a high school dance. Not at weddings, my own or anyone else's.

We're a family of musicians, so the rhythm is easy. It's stepping on his feet I'm worried about. I keep my eyes on our feet for a few moments and graduate to looking at nothing over his shoulder. We move around in a small circle, nothing fancy. My dress sways in time to the music.

The singer swings into the chorus, a memory of a night and a waltz and the sweetheart who was stolen away, crying for all that he's lost.

Dad clears his throat. "Your mother and I went to a dance at Harvard once, at one of the fraternities. A formal, dressy affair. The first dance was a waltz, and I tripped on her dress, and we fell flat." He laughs. "We were famous, or rather, infamous, that evening. We kept dancing, though."

I know what he's thinking, and I know what my line is. It's what I'm supposed to say. I note, with gratitude, that I also want to say it.

"You've kept dancing, more than fifty-five years now." He's done the best he could—I am beginning to feel that, not just say it. When he yelled at Mom, he was afraid that her wandering, a disease symptom, was intentional and meant she was leaving him. As Mom's agitation grew while her ability to reason and understand eroded, as she drifted farther and farther away, as I came in to meddle in the name of "help" and then went away again—always, he was there. He tried, and I tried, and we both have failed in some ways, but he always tried.

"Yup" is all he says. This is the closest we come to apologies. Mom is still sick, and she won't get well, but at least he and I are together again.

The singer repeats the chorus twice, three times, maybe more. I lose count. My heart is full of sorrow, full of the song, its singer forlorn but resigned. His sweetheart is gone. He can't change it. He can only remember, and sing.

One-two-three, *one*-two-three. The sadness in this moment feels just right. It's there, a fact, but there's nothing to do about it. We, too, are at a calm in grief's storm, in Mom's story, in ours. I relax into the dance, caught up in the swirling melody that weaves between and around my father and me.

The singer holds the last note. Still clasping my hand, Dad bows to me. I drop a curtsy, my special dress swishing. Dad leads me back to our seats through what feels like a sea of applause.

Mom watches us, her hand raised in blessing, in benediction. "Perfect," she says.

CURTAIN

9

MEANDER

I look for my mother at the lake every August. I slip away from visiting family to walk the narrow, stony road that my grandfather carved through the woods in the 1930s. Thirty feet above my head, birch leaves whisper. A gull soars by, keening; a crow spits a mocking challenge. Light and shadows, rustlings and silences wrap me in a soft blanket.

This land, with its two small camps on Lake Superior, was her summer home. My mother learned to swim in the shallow bay. She picked blueberries at the top of the cliff that rises, black and solid, from the rocks at the shoreline. She watched thousands of sunrises shoot golden fire across the water, illuminating the contours of Caribou Island on their way.

She died in May of 2000, yet I look for her as I walk the woods. I look for her as I sit at sunrise on the beach, as I row in the bay. I look for her in long midsummer twilights, when the half-cup moon spills a silver path across the water to my feet. I listen for her in the murmur of the birches and breath of the waves. I look for her in the rocks, in the water, in the breeze.

My mother left Port Arthur for Queen's University in the 1930s. She never returned to northwestern Ontario to live full-time, yet she never really left. She wrote the dissertation for her Ph.D. in mathematics at a makeshift desk in the woodshed behind the small camp. After World War II, now married and Jeanne Agnew, she and my father found teaching positions in Oklahoma. She taught in Oklahoma for sixty years. But nothing could sever her connection to this land, this place.

She returned to the lake every summer. August in Oklahoma is severe: acres of shimmering, semi-liquid asphalt reflect thick heat. To escape after the summer term, she packed five kids, a pet or two, and my father into a station wagon and headed north for a few weeks. Like a salmon, she returned every year to the physical place of her beginning—except instead of spawning new offspring, she herself was reborn.

In Oklahoma, Mom ran a disciplined, orderly household. Five children and an active academic career required efficiency.

Life at the lake, though still structured, was more relaxed. As in Oklahoma, we did plenty of chores. Properly supervised, we took turns cooking. My brothers sawed and split logs for the stove and the fireplace. My older sister and I helped my mother wash and dry dishes, beat the rugs, and sweep out the sand tracked inside every day. Mom wasn't exactly a different person at camp—just happier.

My father's primary responsibility, emptying the pails from the outhouse, won him a reprieve from other tasks. Besides, he wasn't an outdoors person. A historian and scholar, not a woodsman, he didn't fix things. He didn't own blue jeans or work boots, didn't use levels and screwdrivers. His tool of choice was a ballpoint pen, applied to paper, driven by his intellect. So he read, scratching notes in margins, or wrote. At the lake, as in Oklahoma, he often preferred to be left alone. It was, after all, his vacation.

And it was our vacation, too. After chores, all of us played, including Mom. One summer when I was seven or so, she and I cobbled together a raft from pulp logs that had escaped the lumber companies' booms and washed up on the beach. Two of my brothers, knee-deep in the frigid water, dragged volleyball-sized rocks into a large pile to serve as a makeshift wharf. My oldest brother spread caulk on all the joints of the old wooden rowboat left over from my grandfather's day, while my sister sketched him.

As Mom and I worked, laying scrap wood across two logs and hammering nails, she told me that the rafts she had made as a child never lasted through the winter. Brushing the silver hair back from her forehead, she watched me pound a nail. The sun warmed our swimsuited bodies, and the morning smelled fresh and new.

"Your Uncle Hugh was much better at it. He'd put four or five or even six logs together and make a huge raft that he could stand up on. Here, lay this one across here. No, like this. See? Okay, nail it. He could pole them across the bay."

"Like the boys last year." I wiped my sweaty palms on my swimsuit and picked up the hammer again. A large raft had turned up on our beach the previous summer. My three older brothers poled it around the point, where the water was ten feet deep. The raft was too dangerous for me to manage, Mom had said. I was too little, not strong or sure enough.

I still wasn't strong enough, not to hammer well, anyway. I was trying, but I must have hit a knot. That nail wasn't going in any farther.

"Yes, like the boys last year. I wonder what happened to that raft over the winter." Mom paused to look out at the water, then shook her head. "Well, as my mother used to say, 'What the lake giveth, the lake taketh away.' Yes, Hugh's rafts were big like that."

I pounded away. A little impatience crept into her voice. "Here, let me."

She took the hammer, and I held the board in place. Meanwhile, I peeked up at her, trying to see the little girl in her lined forehead and greying hair.

She added, "He always had an extra box on them, 'for provisions,' he used to say."

"What's 'provisions'?" I watched her pound fruitlessly at the nail.

"What my mother called 'eats.' Food." She frowned at the nail. "Well, bleah." She drove the shaft of the nail down sideways so it wouldn't stick up and hurt my feet.

I looked at her, eyebrows raised. "Grandma let you take food out on the raft?"

"Oh, no." She tugged on the board to see if it would hold, then handed me another nail. "Here, put it in about there. No, we never had extra food, and besides, we weren't really going anywhere, so we made do with pretend provisions."

She stood up and smiled at our handiwork: two logs, about six inches apart, crossed near one end by three long boards that stuck out like airplane wings. A shorter board, nailed crosswise like the others about halfway back, provided some stability. A masterpiece.

Mom helped me shove the raft the remaining foot or two into the water, and I straddled one of the logs, gasping at the coldwater shock as I sat. I pushed along the lake bottom with my feet until the raft and I were completely free and floating. She watched me for a moment before calling, "Don't go out too far."

"I won't." I only wanted to get out ten yards or so, where the bottom turned to sand. As I kicked and paddled, inching toward my goal, I looked around the small bay. Like the boys, Uncle Hugh had poled rafts past these same black rocks. Meanwhile, my mother had paddled around in the safety of the bay on a smaller craft. Like me.

In August of 2000, three months after my mother died, the family congregated at the lake as usual: my sister and her then-husband, my then-husband and I, my mother's sister, and my father.

One morning during our vacation, I began the job of scraping at the worn, flaking paint on the ancient window frames and walls of our smaller camp, attacking the sickly, too-green yellow with glee. The camp had looked jaundiced for years, and I had selected a warm, brave gold, the colour of the birch leaves in September, to restore it to health, or at least the appearance of it.

The sun, high above the trees, rested warmly on my neck. As I gouged away, tiny flecks of paint showered around me, sticking to my shoulders and hair. Sweat trickled down my backbone, spreading at the waistband of my shorts. The few short balsams between the camp and the lake deflected any breeze from the water.

"Can I help?" Allison, my aunt, asked through the window screen. Her clean white blouse shone in the dim coolness behind the screen. I thought of her arthritic shoulders, her careful, even steps, her seventy-five years.

"No, but thanks." I rested my scraper against the wood and wiped my forehead with the back of my hand. "Hot work."

"But worthy. It's good to see you taking care of the place."

I smiled. It felt good to me, too. When we visited the lake as adults, my mother organized work crews—the price, she said, of vacation. She, not my father, painted the front of the camp this so-wrong colour. But, I told myself, the wan paint was a temporary aberration in the long history of the camp.

So were the years of my mother's illness, which robbed her of her vocabulary and her take-charge personality. But, I reminded myself, those years of her illness were just an aberration, just part of her long life. Still, that vague invalid was the mother I remembered most clearly.

I needed to find the woman she had been. So much I had not been able to control—her illness, her death, the grief. But at least I could fix the colour of the camp. I shifted the scraper in my hand, ready to begin again.

The reflection in the window next to Allison caught my eye. In the old glass, the islands in the bay rippled green and brown against the blue sky and water. I turned to look at them directly. Caribou, the larger island, performed its magic trick, hovering above the surface of the silver-blue water as if unconnected to this world. Just three miles away. But I had never actually touched the island, never set foot on it.

That summer, the first without my mother, I was restless. Watching Caribou wink at me across the water, I thought, *What's there? What could I see?*

As if on cue, our aluminum rowboat glided smoothly around the point into our small bay, steered by our then-husbands and powered by a small rented motor. I caught my breath. It was a calm day, safe enough for a three-mile trip. We could really go to Caribou.

I remembered a conversation with my mother from her last summer. Tired and slightly disoriented after her long day of travel, we'd looked out at Caribou and she'd said, "I don't know if I'm really here or just dreaming that I am."

You're really here, I had said. But where?

Before climbing into the boat, I splashed one double handful of water over my face and another over my head. I settled in and we skimmed over the lake's surface. The droning motor made talking impossible, and I didn't want to talk anyway. The wind cooled my skin and carried away the flecks of scraped paint. The sun caressed my lifted face.

Family inertia. That's my only explanation for vacationing at the lake nearly every summer of my life but never before going those last three miles out to Caribou. Mom had visited the island often in her childhood, in a motorboat her father made by adding a motor he "picked up cheap" at the dump to a wooden rowboat. Sometimes her family— my grandparents, Hugh, Mom, and Allison—spent the day at Caribou, picking raspberries for jam.

That motorboat was long gone by the time I was born. We never had another, and I had never missed having one. The rowboat and occasional rickety raft had always taken me as far as I needed to go. And going out in boats—or watching us row—became a source of fear for Mom as her illness advanced.

But now Mom was gone and I needed to take this trip. I watched Caribou grow on the horizon. A thought dropped into the placid well of my contentment: *If she were still alive and here, we wouldn't be doing this.* I let the wind carry the thought away over the water, ruffled beside me. I looked down beside the boat to admire the clear water darkening, as it deepened, into a cool mallard green.

After a half-hour, Caribou loomed large, its cliff towering over a tree-lined slope. We pulled up along the south side. I hopped out into knee-deep water, bending to rinse my fingers and lift another handful of water to my face. About fifteen feet of beach sloped up steeply in front of me before disappearing into a tangle of evergreens and brush.

I looked back across the water, searching for our camp, even a yellow dot through the trees. Nothing distinguished it from the rest of the shoreline. Turning to the island, I walked up the beach, fighting for balance the whole way. The rocks underfoot had been scoured into smooth spheres by winter upon winter of fierce wind and waves. This side of Caribou bore the brunt of winter storms.

The rocks fascinated me. I picked up one heavy, softball-shaped chunk after another, marvelling. I loaded the pockets of my shorts with speckled stones: dark grey, light grey, nearly white, pink. I already had a favourite, a pink granite oval that fit perfectly into the palm of my hand.

When we were kids, leaving the lake to return to our Oklahoma life was excruciating. The night before we left, we always built a bonfire on the beach. In it, we burned clothes deemed too ragged to bring home. I was half-afraid of fire anyway, and this ritual gave me nightmares. Mom would toss a flannel shirt, still warm from the back of one of my brothers, onto the fire. Through my tears, I'd watch the shirt writhe and twitch, sink onto a log, and disappear into the roaring flames.

The family gathered around a beach fire the summer my mother died, too. My father carefully laid a curl of my mother's hair near the edge of the flames. It caught and burned cleanly. We sang the "Pretty Moon" lullaby that my mother had sung to us as kids, the one my grandmother had sung to my mother and to Allison, the one my oldest brother had sung at my mother's funeral in Oklahoma three months before.

I watched sparks flying upward into the dark evening sky. *Now a piece of Mom is here forever,* I told myself. I tried to feel comforted. Peaceful. But I felt nothing.

Later, the aurora borealis danced turquoise and lime-green in the navy sky, shooting streamers of cool fireworks from behind Caribou. I watched from the beach with my sister, knowing I should be impressed but wanting more.

"It's a cathedral," my sister said. "It's Mom."

"Yes." I said it only because I knew she wanted me to. I still wanted my mother back, the mother I had before the disease made her forget her home.

Since then, time and the world have brought the peace I wanted that evening. The three-mile trip to Caribou was only the first leg on a longer journey. My marriage, already weak, collapsed under the weight of my grief. I left a life that never fit me.

Now, I sit at my desk, holding my granite egg from Caribou and thinking of my mother. I press the stone firmly between my palms and rest it against my lips. It smells wild and old and clean. I close my eyes and picture huge waves hurling my rock up the beach. I watch my rock roll back toward the water only to be grabbed and thrown again, time after time—in my time, in my mother's time before me, in her mother's time before her.

I hear the lake's music. A loon whistles in the pre-dawn grey. Waves gently tease pebbles from the beach. The wind swirls through the birches.

At my desk, I lift my eyes and see Caribou itself across the water. I look for my mother at the lake each summer because I know she is here. She is home. And so am I.

10

ALL I CAN SAY

Let mortals beware
Of words, for
With words we lie
W. H. Auden, "A Hymn to the United Nations"

I never expected there would be music at this funeral.

Before Eric begins, he apologizes to the thirty of us gathered in the pet cemetery. "Sorry, I don't know music," he says. "But I played for Fancy. We did this together. So I want to do it now. I'm sorry if the music isn't good."

He sits cross-legged beside his dog's body and breathes gently into a harmonica. A thin line of notes meanders upward, ruffling the leaves on the trees that protect us, the mourners, from the slanting late-afternoon sun. We file past the sleeping bag where Fancy lies, surrounded by her toys, framed photos, and flowers. Eric inhales and exhales. The random notes wind around and among us, a cord that binds us in grief.

Eric claims not to know music because he is culturally Deaf. The notes he plays are random in part because he can't hear them. Fancy was his service dog. When he apologizes for not knowing music, he doesn't use his voice. Instead, he communicates in American Sign Language, his hands and arms flowing in concert with the expressions passing across his face. His right fist rubs a quick circle on his chest, his index finger brushes his chest, his fingertips touch his forehead and then open as his head shakes, his open right palm waves in the crook of his left elbow. The signs for SORRY, I, DON'T-KNOW, and MUSIC.

I blink away the tears to keep my eyes clear so that I can hear him. But I also listen at a deeper level—in my body.

My most vivid memory from my mother's funeral service is also the music. My oldest brother sang a family lullaby. Only then did another brother's composed façade crack, his shoulders shuddering in a sob under his tweed coat. He shook his head and pinched the bridge of his nose to stop his tears. I rubbed his shoulder, happy to cry real tears after crying invisibly during the years of Mom's illness.

My mother's illness taught me about communicating without a shared spoken language. As she lost words, I interpreted her feelings and guessed her needs from her tone of voice and gestures instead of the gibberish her mouth produced. I sat with her and followed her gaze, commenting on what I thought she might be looking at. To make her laugh, I laughed.

We also connected through music. In her last year, she had seizures and moved into a nursing home. Her first weekend there, my sister and I sat with her at the piano in the institution's dining room. The three of us played easy duets from a book my sister and I had used decades before. My sister provided the foundation in the bass while my mother and I played the melody in different octaves.

My mother played more accurately than I did. Even in the nursing home, she could still follow the line of notes across the page. But after a few minutes, she lost momentum. Her hands dropped into her lap, and she sat motionless between us, her "girls." Her smile lingered a few minutes longer, then it, too, faded.

Throughout her illness, my mother could make me understand her. She spent her last Christmas in the hospital, fighting pneumonia. Her eyes, ice-blue and sharp above the oxygen tube snaking into her nose, snapped at me in fear, in command. I stood at the foot of the bed, facing her directly. In that frigid winter hospital room, I felt her wishes in my body as tangibly as if I'd walked into a wall of hot, humid summer air. *I hurt. Make it stop. Ease my breathing.*

Two years later, Eric became my American Sign Language teacher for one semester. At the end of the term, he teased me about having been a serious person, sombre and closed off to him and my classmates earlier in the semester.

I protested, as much as my limited ASL vocabulary allowed. "No!" I exclaimed, my index and middle fingers snapping against my thumb to show my vehemence. "Never! I'm shy; I'm scared. But my heart and mind were never closed!"

"Yes," he insisted, "I got bad vibes." His brown eyes laughed as he fingerspelled "vibes" for me; he raised an eyebrow to be sure I understood before going on. "Then after three, maybe four weeks, you opened up. I thought, 'Finally!'"

I rolled my eyes and signed, "No! Never closed. Just shy, nervous, scared."

His fist nodded "yes" at me again. "Whatever," I responded, recognizing "Did not!" "Did too!" from arguments with my brothers.

Eric believed that learning ASL had forced me to become more expressive and direct. Later, I decided he was right—but only half-right. ASL had reminded me of something I'd learned before. It was my mother's illness that had first taught me how to listen to ideas and feelings with my body, searching for meaning without always assigning words. But when my mother died, I had been relieved to be able to retreat into words. To hide behind them. To use them—as I refused to use alcohol, drugs, or religion—to anesthetize my pain.

During the first year after her death, I searched for an image that would perfectly describe the desolation I felt. Trudging through a desert. Trekking the windswept, ice-covered Arctic. Slogging in quicksand. I desperately wanted to capture that feeling in words, to fence it in. If I could find the perfect metaphor, the pain of grief would lose its power. I would be its master.

The hurt would go away.

At Fancy's funeral, Eric stands tall and pale in a yellow cotton shirt and tan slacks. A brown seed necklace lies on his chest. He had been battered and bruised when the drunk driver hit his van and killed Fancy, just four days earlier, and he will need back surgery. However, he moves through the warm June afternoon without apparent effort, his thoughts and attention on Fancy.

He says, "Some people don't think animals have souls. I believe animals have souls and spirits, the same as people."

Eric is a large man, a broad-shouldered man—and a Deaf man. He can be intimidating to hearing people. Fancy, a medium-sized terrier mix with laughing eyes and black fur that floated with her prancing walk, helped break the ice. Her friendly presence made it easier for people to connect to Eric. Fancy also taught Eric about the hearing world—he learned about people from watching the way they treated her. Of course, Fancy worked for him: she protected him, alerting him to a ringing doorbell or telephone, to a stranger's presence. But Fancy also kept him company. Loved him.

Eric says, "She touched many people's lives, the lives of you here today and the lives of other people who said they couldn't be here."

As he speaks in ASL, Debbie is his voice for the hearing world. A professional interpreter for eleven years, she still has trouble keeping up with him at times. She waves gently in the air, and he backs up to repeat his last statement. She's not only his interpreter—she and her husband are Eric's friends. Eric had been driving home from working on their farm when the accident happened. Debbie, too, had known and loved Fancy.

When I listen with my ears, I find the funeral oddly quiet, compared to a church funeral. No booming organ, no choral music, no histrionic sobs. Just sparrows cheeping as they swoop past. A few cars and trucks murmur on the state highway a mile away. The tags on Fancy's chain collar, which Eric has tied to his necklace, sometimes clink as Eric signs. Otherwise, the only sounds are muffled sniffles from people in the group, whimpers from a dog friend of Fancy's, and Debbie's voice.

But when I listen with my body, the funeral is very loud. I shut out Debbie's words to hear Eric in the way my mother and Eric taught me. If communicating with my mother in that hospital room was like walking into a wall of hot air, listening to Eric is a little like standing in the blast of a fire hose. I must lean into it merely to remain upright.

"I don't have anger toward the driver who did this," Eric says. For "anger," his hands, fingers spread and bent like claws, jerk from the centre of his sternum upward to his shoulders. Surely it would be normal for him to be angry, for his rage to explode in violence, like the sign, like a volcano. But he continues, "It's not good to live angry. It's important to forgive."

Grief is a land of opposites. I never felt more alone than when my mother died, but her illness and death also made me part of a new community. My wounded heart opened to others' losses. When other people mentioned death and grief, I listened and asked questions so they could talk. Because of grief's shadows on my soul, the beauty I could see—green leaves on trees, a smile passed to a friend—appeared brighter. Grief carved out more room for gratitude and forgiveness.

At the same time, grief isolated me. I lived far away from the other members of my family. My then-husband hadn't known my mother before her illness and was wrapped up in grief of his own. No one around me needed to reminisce about my mother, to conjure up the woman she had been before her illness. A few people who knew of her death murmured a condolence and changed the subject. Others knew and said nothing, as if my grief could infect them or cause their family members to die. Sometimes I looked in the mirror for the mark on my forehead, the one that must brand me as someone grieving, someone to be shunned.

On bad days, I could feel a dark hand closing around my heart. I could be doing something as simple as shopping when the hand clenched. Mothers and daughters looking for summer sandals, trying on flip-flops and laughing together—my envy made it difficult for me even to breathe.

The people who did talk to me were full of advice, of talk. They had little interest in listening. Listening might lead to tears—mine, theirs.

In my grief, I didn't have a person to forgive, as Eric did. But I did need to learn how to live in the world again.

Time helped. I wrote, went to a support group, played music, sang, cried, laughed, and wrote some more. I felt joy again, on occasion. I became interested in the world beyond myself. I enrolled in an American Sign Language class.

And I later understood that my wounds scarred over in part because I had covered over that part of me that had learned to hear with my body, below the code of words. I needed the protection the scars gave me to get through the world day by day.

In ASL class, Eric pushed me to open myself again. He reached for every person in that class at a deep level. He butted into our beginner conversations, sparse in vocabulary but full of earnest struggle to express ourselves. He teased, he poked, he challenged. He told us over and over that ASL is not fluttering hands making signs that correspond to English words. Instead, ASL is a unique language. Adverbs, adjectives, and other parts of speech appear in movements of the face, arms, and the whole body.

Periodically, Eric gave us pep talks. "Practise hard, and you will learn better and better and better. Then if you see a Deaf kid, you can go up to him and chat with him. He'll be excited."

As I studied ASL, I began to relearn that words are simply tools. To communicate with another person, in any language, I must open myself to be touched. I must stretch myself to understand.

Eric likes to make people laugh. At Fancy's funeral he lays a pair of socks near Fancy because she loved to steal his clean socks and run outside with them. We muster a smile at the story. Eric leads a final prayer, then kneels again. He lays his face next to Fancy's and says softly but clearly, with his voice, "I love you, Fancy."

Two of his friends pick up the framed photos and wrap her body in the sleeping bag. A staff member from the pet cemetery helps lower the bundle into the waiting hole. We mourners stand quietly, taking the moment to breathe or to wipe our faces.

I watch Eric. I see him slip his harmonica into the grave with Fancy. As I wait in the receiving line to speak with him, I cry again for the simple lament he played earlier, notes now buried. I know, as he cannot yet, that he will feel like playing music again. I want to tell him that, and more: Sit bravely in the darkness. Watch for the sunrise. Care for yourself, carefully. Let grief change you, because it will anyway, and you shouldn't fight its changes.

When it's my turn, I step forward and stand on tiptoe to pull his tall, broad body to me. His arms wrap my shoulders in a warm circle, and I feel him draw a breath. A final squeeze, and we let go.

That's all I can say. And all I need to.

11

THE HOUSE THAT BROKE MY HEART

One morning in late July of 2004, I loaded a suitcase into the trunk of my Camry. I don't remember scratching the dogs' ears, though I know I did. I don't remember saying good-bye to my husband. He might have been working at his company's office that day, but still, we would have said good-bye—wouldn't we? Whatever our leave-taking, I do know that our eyes didn't meet. We'd long ago stopped searching out the other's gaze.

I backed out, sitting in the driveway to be sure the garage door closed fully. The perfectly nice split-level house had plenty of room. Each of us had a home office. My husband's office held stacks of paper, musical instruments, and computer equipment. I'd filled mine with memorabilia from Lake Superior—chunks of amethyst, birchbark baskets, watercolours of lake and birch forest scenes, photos of the aurora borealis in winter. I loved working surrounded by these talismans of our summer camps, faint copies of reality but better than nothing.

We'd become experts at being alone under the same roof.

I wound through the city streets, eventually heading north on I-25, toward Cheyenne. Ahead of me lay the nearly 2000 kilometres of my annual trek to our family place on Lake Superior. I looked forward to a few weeks with my father and sister, who were flying in after I'd been there several days to clean and ready both camps. But I welcomed the two full days of driving. By myself. With myself.

For the first hour, mountains rose to my left; to my right, cattle-dotted rangeland stretched to a far horizon. Keeping me company, the minutiae of leave-taking: Did the car have gas enough to get into Wyoming, where a fill-up would be less expensive? Did I have enough cash for water and snacks along the way? Could I reach my rain jacket in case of afternoon thundershowers?

By the time I reached Cheyenne and turned East onto I-80, those concerns had floated away and other thoughts surfaced. With the mountains fading to a dark line in my rear-view mirror, and nothing but flat Nebraska ahead, optimism surged through my arms into my hands. I recognized how pleased and free I felt—how thrilling it was to leave home.

Or perhaps I wasn't leaving home. Perhaps I was going home, to this place I loved so much.

"What do you want to be when you grow up?" From about the age of eight, I'd answer with my choice of the moment—veterinarian, engineer, historian, librarian, psychologist, neurologist. Then I'd add, "And move to Canada and live at the lake year-round."

I wasn't made for summers in Oklahoma. In July, temperatures climb to more than 100 degrees Fahrenheit, bubbling the tar that patched the cracks of our concrete streets. On especially warm days, I'd stand in front of an air conditioner vent and dream of running along our sand-and-pebble beach, a breeze off the water of Lake Superior ruffling my hair.

My mother also loved being at the lake in the summer. But when I talked about living there all year, she warned me about two things: the expense of maintaining the property, and the difficulties of winter. On an Oklahoma summer day, the piles of snow and ice she described sounded heavenly, if completely foreign to my experience. And as for the money? With the confidence of childhood, I'd shrug. Somehow, I'd be able to handle all that. My life would work out.

Since my mother's death in 2000, I'd avoided making big decisions as my immediate two-person/two-dog family weathered several losses. While I walked in the pale world that no longer included my mother, my husband grieved his father, who'd died unexpectedly a few months earlier.

We slogged through the days. Activities that had once brought us together, from performing music to playing with our dogs, lost their appeal. The silence between us grew.

A year after my mother's death, I'd taken a class in American Sign Language in a search for something interesting to do. I'd fallen in love with the visual requirements of the language. To communicate with each other, we had to look each other in the face to take in the unity of hand and body movements, along with facial expressions. I'd never felt as seen as I had while trying to communicate in ASL. Intense, immersive study group sessions and socials with the Deaf community left me energized, but with even less interest in my husband and his version of silence, whatever it meant—indifference, perhaps jealousy.

To take advanced ASL classes, I'd enrolled in a two-year college program in interpreting. The first year had ended in May, and I'd considered quitting the program. Although I still loved the language, I didn't want to become an interpreter—I had enough trouble communicating with people myself to take on a role facilitating communication for others.

In the car, I sighed. I hated to leave ASL, but it wasn't fair to take on a role I didn't want. Another dead end. So many of them behind me.

Nebraska interstate thrummed under my car's tires at eighty miles per hour. Although I stopped myself from making yet another extensive catalogue of my losses, my husband's perceived failings, and my own, the highway sounds couldn't drown out the echo of my husband's reproaches. Especially the one repeated most often: "I don't feel close to you."

Sometimes I'd ignored it—surely that was just a momentary thing, a fleeting feeling, something you say and later regret.

Other times, I'd ask, "How can I change that?"

His response: "You can't."

I'd shrug and wish away the pain—his and mine both—by doing something constructive, like laundry or work.

But as I sped across Nebraska, nearing Iowa, my eyes widened. I sat up straighter behind the wheel and gripped it firmly.

I wasn't listening. I wasn't hearing my husband.

He said he didn't feel close to me. He said I couldn't make it better.

I blinked tears away and looked for a safe place to pull over. At a rest area, I turned off the ignition but sat in the car, stunned.

I hadn't listened. But I should.

Perhaps I should respect him enough to believe him.

Other questions took my breath away. I got out of the car and paced up and down the sidewalk.

Did I feel close to him? No. Had I tried to bridge the space between us? Yes, I'd kept reaching out into that ever-widening gap. But I'd grown tired.

Did I still want to save our marriage? No.

I waited for more tears. Instead, my sadness cleared. Somewhere, deep down, I'd already known.

So, what was I waiting for?

Back in the car on the highway, I wondered what my mother would advise. "Make a decision and make the best of it," probably. She was always impatient with my dithering.

Perhaps I'd done that—perhaps I'd made the best of this marriage. I'd certainly tried, for years. And it no longer served either of us.

Maybe it was time for a new decision, new action, something bigger than laundry or work. Could I leave? Did I really have to return to what I thought of as "my regular life" in that perfectly nice house?

My heart started to beat faster. Freelance writing, my work, was completely portable. My time learning ASL seemed to be over. Could I finally do it—chase my childhood dream?

At least I'd picked the perfect time to consider my options. I had hours in front of me to mull it over. And my destination was the place where my life had always made sense, even after my mother's death. There, I could focus on the small, satisfying tasks that supported everyday life, like feeding the fire in the wood stove, reminding myself to stop skimping on small twigs. I could commune with myself through the years as I lay in bed, watching the night gather through the windows, rippled with time. I could talk with my sister, either rowing together on the big lake or walking the path back and forth to the big camp for meals and chats with my father.

I'd sift through possibilities. I might even find a way to tackle all the big responsibilities of our property, the ones Mom had always handled. Since her death, they'd felt beyond my ability to address.

Somewhere near the Nebraska-Iowa border, I set aside what I was leaving behind and looked forward to what I'd find when I arrived.

Changes had come to our camp property in the years since I'd declared my intention to live there year-round someday. Oh, the essentials remained: two rustic structures facing separate bays, beautiful locations on a lovely lake. But now, a large house loomed between them.

In the summer of 1984, looking ahead to her retirement, my mother wanted to make the larger camp a more comfortable place to stay the whole summer. She wanted to have the camp re-roofed and electricity installed, which would enable indoor plumbing and hot water in a small bathroom addition.

Selling land to finance these improvements made logical sense. Logic, the world in which Mom operated best. The two camps sat at opposite ends of approximately ten wooded acres. The middle section of land, which tended to be boggy anyway, could lift out easily without disturbing the privacy of either camp.

When Mom told us she'd arranged to sell it, she listed the advantages of the sale, adding, "You kids won't be able to afford it when I'm gone anyway."

Her lack of faith in my childhood fantasy broke my heart. I was as furious as any immature twenty-three-year-old could be. I was also defensive. Mom was right, and I didn't like it. My bachelor's degree qualified me for receptionist work making barely more than minimum wage. My siblings had families and their own dreams to support. All five of us put together couldn't have bought that section of land from her.

I took out my anger on the new house. During the two years that the new owners took out trees, filled in marshy areas with dirt, and built a large, modern home between our camps, I resented the changes on principle.

Even when the owners had their young children write letters to Mom, illustrating their delight at living by the lake, I was annoyed—they lived my dream.

Eventually, even I had to acknowledge the upsides to Mom's improvements. A warm shower at camp was far superior to cold-water baths in the lake. The phone line meant we could stay in touch more easily—no more trips to town or a gas station to make long-distance phone calls.

As the years passed and I recognized my parents' happiness in their improved camp, my resentment faded. My eyes got used to the house's presence on the shoreline—I stopped thinking of it as a "monstrosity" and a "scar on the landscape." The original owners sold the home to a nice couple with teenagers.

This couple, Roy and Phyllis, proved to be excellent neighbours, far more interested in watching wildlife in the reeds along their shoreline than trucking in sand for a beach. They, too, preferred canoes to powerboats or jet skis. About once a year, my parents had dessert and coffee with them. Although younger than my mother, Phyllis too taught mathematics, and she and Mom talked shop.

Over time, my father and Roy took on similar roles. Mom's Alzheimer's became more pronounced each year. Phyllis's MS also worsened. Mom died in 2000. Phyllis died in 2002, though we didn't know it until we received Roy's Christmas card. That summer, my father had been unable to shake a lung infection. Though he'd come to the lake as usual, we saw few people and had thought nothing of Roy's absence.

We were all saddened at Phyllis's passing. We'd miss her cheerful, intelligent presence. So many changes, so many losses. What would be next? With Phyllis gone and his children grown, would Roy want to sell his home and move into a smaller place? And what about my father's health—it had stabilized after that difficult summer. But how many years would he have left? What would happen to our property then?

Every year, before I left our camps to return to "my regular life" in that "perfectly nice house" in the U.S., I'd walk down to the beach. "Someday," I'd whisper. "Someday, I won't have to leave."

Every year, I made that promise—to myself? To the camp? To the lake? I was never sure. And the logistics remained complete fantasy.

All across Iowa, surrounded by cornfields even after turning left at Des Moines to head north on I-35, I thought about the summer ahead.

Every year, I tried to do one maintenance chore. The handyman who put in the water lines and kept trees off the road wasn't able, physically, to do much more. We couldn't afford to hire people for painting or roofing, even if we magically knew what needed to be done, and in what order. How would we know who was trustworthy? How could we evaluate estimates in the two or three weeks we were there?

The bigger camp where my father stayed was likely in reasonably good shape. I'd open the windows, sweep it thoroughly, and wash down the kitchen and bedding. Unless I found other signs of invasion, whether wasps in the eaves or squirrels in the attic, we'd be good to go once I stocked the kitchen. The smaller camp desperately needed some structural work, which was far beyond my ability even to evaluate. However, it also needed a coat of paint inside—that was more my speed. Maybe painting would be my summer project.

I wondered about trees growing up elsewhere on the property, especially over footpaths. Maybe Roy would teach me to use his chainsaw. The previous summer, we'd found a tree that had fallen directly into the bay near our smaller camp. My sister and I had asked Roy for help, and he'd dispatched it into neat piles of brush and wood along the shore. To repay him, we'd invited him to dinner, cooking local fish. Dinner conversation included Canadian politics. We found he was only a few years older than my oldest brother.

My sister had asked to borrow his computer so she could check email. While Sue was occupied in the den, he and I sat in the main room overlooking the lake and made small talk—never my strong suit. Luckily, Roy and I had plenty in common. We discussed the history of the English language, especially the differences between Middle and Old English. He recited parts of *Beowulf* and Anglo-Saxon religious poetry. I asked him about winter, and after talking about his snow blower, he described skiing over the frozen bay to the islands. He told me about deer—does with fawns in the spring, young bucks sparring in the fall, and their footprints through January's snowdrifts. How everything is the same every year, and also different. He asked about my mother and the family, the camps and their history. We discussed writing, a little, about which no one else in my life showed any curiosity.

There in the car heading north on I-35 through Minnesota, I remembered that Roy's family had owned a camp across the bay. I wondered what he knew about structural engineering. Perhaps he could advise me about the leaking roof and sagging rooms at our little camp. Perhaps I could overcome family inertia enough to do some research. I might not be able to fix everything, but I could at least find out what we could do to keep the camp from collapsing in on itself.

I pushed beyond Minneapolis, driving more than fourteen hours that first day. I lay awake in my Spartan motel room. My body thrummed from the car's movement. A voice kept whispering in my ear: Is it time? Can I move?

The next day, that voice kept me company as cornfields gave way to poplars and pines, which were in turn replaced by birch and balsam. Shelves of granite peeked through the grass of the highway median, and finally, I drove over the hill at Duluth. The sun sparkled on Lake Superior in welcome. I hummed as I sped along the north shore, crossed the border, and finally arrived at our place.

Three weeks later, I drove my Camry in the other direction. On my way south to Duluth, I looked for real estate signs—maybe I'd live in Minnesota while I figured out how to emigrate. If freelancing didn't work for some reason, I could do anything, even get another job answering phones. To fill in gaps, I could cash in an investment I'd made with money my mother had left me. I could think of no better reason or time to use it.

At the last Lake Superior lookout, I said good-bye, but promised both the lake and myself that I'd be back—and soon.

South through Minnesota and Iowa to I-80, I marvelled at the past weeks. I'd asked Roy for help seeing what needed to be done. He'd walked through our smaller camp, looking closely at the piano falling into the floor in the back corner, at the sloping floor of the front room, at the eavestroughs directing rainwater into the foundations.

I'd braced myself in case he said what I'd feared for years: "It's not worth saving. Time to sell this place or tear it down."

Instead, Roy had run his hand down some of the interior walls, recognizing boxcar panelling from grain cars. He'd admired the stone fireplace in the corner, built from rocks picked up along the shore.

He'd seen what I'd seen.

His verdict: "It's all doable. The work might take a few years, but it's possible to make this place sound again."

He'd bought dinner, picking up Chinese food in town. We sat at his kitchen table, looking out onto the bay where I'd rowed for a half-hour that very morning before cleaning out the back kitchen at the big camp. The eastern sky glowed pink as the sun set behind us. The water calmed and turned to quicksilver.

"You take on a lot of responsibility," he'd said. "Remember when I took out that tree last year? You looked so sad."

"I couldn't stop thinking about all I wish I could do, and how little time I have to do any of it before I have to go home again. I still feel that." I sighed and looked down at my plate.

"What are you going home to?" His voice was quiet, but I knew he looked at me. "I don't need an answer, but maybe you do." He picked up our plates. "How's your writing going?"

I just shook my head, and we changed the subject to bats and hummingbirds, ravens and gulls.

The next morning, Roy left for a long weekend with golfing buddies. I'd gone for a row, as usual. In the middle of the big bay, I stopped to lean on the oars. I looked for the kitchen windows, where we'd sat the previous evening. Had that conversation really happened, at that kitchen table in that bay window? In that house? THAT house? In the house I'd hated and resented and come only grudgingly to accept? Yes. Roy had seen me. He'd heard me.

I turned west on I-80 toward Nebraska and Colorado. The Rocky Mountains grew in front of me. I knew I wasn't going home, only to the place I happened to live. I'd have tearful conversations, make difficult plans, pack boxes, and leave behind the life I'd known there, to return north and east, to my home at the lake.

I didn't know all the steps, yet—all the highways and byways that lay ahead of me. But I knew I could figure them out. I'd made this decision, and I'd make the best of it. I hoped Mom would be proud.

A few months later, I was living in a Thunder Bay apartment with a view of Lake Superior. I had only a tourist visa and left again before Christmas to spend time with my father and sister. It took months of research and paperwork to stay permanently.

Throughout it all, Roy and I sat at other tables and shared other meals. We stood on his deck, looking at the same view. His steady presence buoyed me when the logistics of moving and immigrating weighed on my heart. At last, I noticed that I talked over every decision with him. That when I looked at him, he was already looking at me. That his blue eyes held laughter and curiosity and respect. I reached out my hand, and he took it. And held on.

I knew that in Roy, I'd found someone with whom I could admire Lake Superior's mornings and evenings. Someone who could skip stones better than I did. A partner to support my writing and teach me to use a chainsaw. Someone with whom I could see and be seen, hear and be heard.

Sometimes it felt as if he'd been waiting for me, choosing to stay in the beautiful place he loved. Mom's property sale had made it all possible.

We married in August of 2007, and now I live year-round in the house that broke my heart—and made it whole again.

12

SAGUARO

I.

On his first trip to Tucson in 2005, Roy marvelled at the landscape, so different from our view in Northwestern Ontario.

"I can't tell what I'm looking at. I don't know what's an abandoned vacant lot and what's xeriscaped, or a garden, that's meant to look that way."

To me, Arizona looked familiar. I'd often visited my sister, Sue, sometimes with my parents. We'd gone to museums and done other typical tourist things. After my mother died, my father and I continued to rendezvous there with Sue, usually in the spring.

Roy's comment made me really study Tucson for the first time in years.

Against the desert's thirst-inducing shades of brown, the dusty greens of stumpy trees and shrubs invited food names—olive and sage and artichoke and avocado. Most of the growth hunched close to the earth, but saguaro cacti towered twenty or more feet tall, with "arms" pointing sideways, up, and down. Impressive enough up close, they were large enough to appear like stubble on faraway hillsides.

Occasionally, I'd seen saguaros sporting a bristling white cap of spines, with blossoms, and with fruit. But I'd grown accustomed to them.

More than a decade later, I'm still grateful for Roy's comment. I looked at Tucson in a new way, and I saw my father with new eyes.

II.

Water is such a visible part of our lives at home. Lake Superior's steel-blue waves pound the beach during autumn and spring storms, rounding pebbles and polishing driftglass. Roy has spent nearly all his life on the Canadian Shield, amid lakes, rivers, and muskeg swamps teeming with life. It's a landscape of obvious plenty, even where the granite lies beneath only a foot or two of soil.

We watch water at work in the birches. In late May, they form chartreuse buds that open and spread into kelly-green leaves in June, droop in emerald rags in late August, and shower like new loonies in early October.

Even winter's palette—blues and greys for water and sky, butter and silver for sun and snow and ice—conveys life and movement. We've learned to look for it and love it, too.

But different people love different landscapes. My father had never really enjoyed our family camps on Lake Superior, not the way my mother and the rest of us had. I wasn't sure that he'd continue coming up after Mom died. But he insisted.

In the years between Mom's death and my move to Canada, Sue and I came to the lake when he did. Late mornings, we'd show up at the big camp and walk with him to the little camp for time on the beach and lunch. Mid-afternoon, he'd walk back alone. We'd follow later to make our family supper there.

Through the years, we drove between the camps in rain or if time pressed. Occasionally he'd be tired and we'd drive to accommodate his lungs. By the summer of 2006, driving had become the unspoken norm. He made the walk only twice—slowly, with my company. Just to prove to himself, and to me, that he still could.

III.

In 2007, my father and I met Sue in Tucson for our usual March vacation. But my father was tired when he left Oklahoma, and in Arizona, he continued to find breathing difficult—a worrying indication of a lung infection complicating his chronic heart and lung disease.

We took him to the hospital on the Ides of March. Early in the morning on his third day, he went into cardiac arrest. Sue and I caught up to him in the Coronary ICU, where he was sedated and on a respirator. We wanted to stay with him, in case his condition changed. But once we were in his room, we had nothing to do other than look at his ninety-year-old unconscious body and worry.

Around us, machines beeped and flashed, their tubes and hoses his lifelines. Fluids and air: pushed in, drawn out. Numbers and lines in neon colours—blue and yellow, mostly; occasionally orange or red—flashed and crawled across screens.

I didn't know what information was important. Which beeps were alarms, which were mere notifications, and which indicated a continued status quo? I had no way to tell.

In that room, I didn't know where it was okay to sit, to stand, to lean, to leave my purse. In the swirling emotions of that moment, I didn't know how to read the room's landscape.

IV.

My father was born during the Great War, in Illinois, the Land of Lincoln. He was one of a cluster of six children, his parents a schoolteacher and a country doctor. He was named for his father and called "Junior." His parents' expectations for him were high, and he grew up with a finely honed sense of duty.

At an early age, Dad became fascinated with history. He memorized facts about presidents and vice-presidents, their cabinet members and their major accomplishments, and hectored his three younger brothers into "playing school" until they rebelled: "Junior, nobody cares about your old presidents!"

My father's family had more children than money, even before the Great Depression arrived with Dad's adolescence. Early on, he became acquainted with "making do" and "taking care," with measuring and saving. He spread a thin skim of jam or butter—never both—on toast. The big ball of broken shoestrings, saved during his childhood and teenage years "because they might be useful someday," waited patiently in the top dresser drawer in the bedroom of his family home for forty years, until he and his siblings assembled for their mother's funeral.

By the time I knew him, my father had become a history professor. He knew everything—I inherited this belief from my older siblings—but he never answered our questions, pointing us instead to the encyclopedia: "Look it up in the *World Book*."

My parents were both forty-three when I was born. I have only a few memories of my father from my preschool years, but I know he was there—in the air, taken for granted, as middle-class parents could be in the middle of North America in the mid-twentieth century.

Photos of my father and me from my early years show him standing behind me, one or both of his hands on my shoulders, in connection and restraint.

V.

In the summer of 2006, my father readied himself to return to Oklahoma after his two-week stay at the lake. He pulled his suit jacket over his long-sleeved dress shirt and the stooped shoulders beneath, checked his shirt pocket for pens, and patted the coat's pockets for his spiral-bound calendar. He chose slip-on leather shoes more convenient for going through security at airports, instead of the white tennis shoes he'd adopted in recent years.

He looked around. His suitcase was packed, but he wasn't ready to leave.

"I'd like to go to the other camp again."

We drove the half-mile. Security against bears, we told each other, but we both knew we were really securing his breath and heartbeat and strength against the rest of his day—ten hours of travel.

At the beach, we settled into chairs. The insistent choppy waves made just enough noise to prevent small talk. And anyway, neither of us felt the need to fill silences.

Our arrival startled a herring gull into takeoff. Small but full-grown, it had shed the dull brownish-grey of immaturity for smart white, with black accents. It hung twenty feet above us, nearly motionless. To ride the invisible currents, it made minute adjustments, tiny contractions and expansions in its black-barred wingspan. Then it rolled onto its side and dove headfirst toward the water, slapped the surface with its feet, and popped back up again. No fish. It drifted back up to its invisible perch.

My father and I watched the bird, and I also watched my father. I thought about what I'd learned to see.

VI.

I am four or five years old. Daddy lets me watch him shave. I stand in the bathroom doorway. I can see him and also, sometimes, his reflection in the small medicine-cabinet mirror. He points his chin up. With a long-bristled brush, his slim fingers curled around the knobby handle, he works white lather across his neck and face. For a brief moment, he looks like Santa Claus.

He runs hot water—just a trickle—and holds his razor underneath it. Then he scrapes the razor down his face once. He returns the razor to the stream to clear the dark-flecked foam before scraping again.

In the white layer, long strips of his cheeks appear, then his neck and chin, and finally his upper lip. He wipes his face and ears with a damp towel and finishes with slaps of Aqua Velva on his cheeks, and then he again looks and smells like the Daddy I know.

He shaves every day, even—perhaps especially—on Christmas morning. He insists on his daily routine of breakfast and shaving before we are allowed to see the tree and open presents. We five kids quarrel and squirm while we wait.

VII.

At home, Roy and I are captive to and captivated by Lake Superior's moods and power. Waves brought sand to cover the clay deposits in the bay in front of us. Water throws pebbles against rocks and rocks against boulders, rounding edges and reshaping the basalt cliffs beside us.

Water has always been here. Nine thousand years ago, water as ice carved ruts into the granite shoreline. In winter, water falls from the sky to lie on the ground as snow and ice before relenting in the spring to melt and soak into the soil and moss.

When Roy and I visit Sue, his questions about geology send me to online encyclopaedias, where I read about water throughout Arizona's history. During the Cambrian Period, a shallow sea covered central North America. The walls of the Grand Canyon, just 350 miles north of Tucson, cradle jellyfish fossils.

Water has always been there, too—ever-present, if invisible.

VIII.

During my school years, Dad seemed always to be in one of two places: sequestered in his study or frowning at the evening news on the television in the family room. Mom usually sent me to call him to supper, and he'd growl at the interruption before slamming down his clipboard or book and drifting to the table, where the rest of us waited.

Mealtimes consisted of variations on meat-plus-starch-plus-vegetable, along with formal conversation that ignored my father's snappish temper. When I was finally excused from the table, I'd escape to chores or homework or books, but I couldn't escape the atmosphere of gloom.

That's why, when I was in my twenties and casting about for direction in life, I was surprised to find my father a mild and steady presence while my mother lectured and prodded and found fault, in her usual way. I began to wonder why I'd irritated my father so much when I was younger.

The encyclopedia reminded me of the turmoil of the late 1960s through the mid-1970s: the war in Viet Nam, the assassinations of Robert F. Kennedy and Martin Luther King, Jr., the "summer of love" that all parents found bewildering.

In those years, my father was in his fifties. As academic theories changed, he felt alienated from his university's history department. But possibly the most important events for him all related to Nixon: the Watergate break-in, Nixon's disgraceful re-election, the investigation, his unwilling resignation, and his eventual pardon by Gerald Ford.

No wonder my father—the Navy veteran of the Second World War, the devotee of social order and routine and institutions, the lover of history's great figures, the idolizer of American presidents—was annoyed so much of that time. What a relief to see that I hadn't necessarily caused all of his irritation.

Fortunately, my father had also found the United Methodist Church, an institution that welcomed and nurtured his gifts. His involvement there, along with his hopefulness, increased about the time I graduated from high school. It helped create the gentle man who later supported me.

IX.

I'd always thought of my mother as the practical one. Though she loved an elegant mathematical proof, she also maintained an interest in the ways mathematics could be applied. My father's interests seemed more hypothetical—church politics and governance, for example. But sometimes he surprised me with observations of the ways big ideas affected daily life.

On a flight to Tucson together, I watched our plane's shadow sweep from Oklahoma City toward the Texas Panhandle.

He motioned to the window. "Roosevelt's New Deal, writ large."

Puzzled, I looked down from 30,000 feet at what looked like metal insects perched in circles of green among reddish-greyish-brownish rectangles of land. "You mean the irrigation?"

"Yes. See, every farm has a pond, too. The Soil Conservation Service did that. It was a state program, but it grew out of Roosevelt's agricultural relief programs. To be sure Oklahoma would never suffer another Dust Bowl."

Another summer afternoon in Oklahoma, he asked me to shop for clothes with him. The men's store in downtown Stillwater was having a sale, and he said he needed my advice. He tried on several pairs of slacks in shades of sand, dark brown, and olive. He refused to buy the practical khaki ones I advocated for.

"I had enough of that colour in the war." He chose the dark olive ones and changed the subject.

He'd never mentioned that, not once, in the four decades I'd known him. He'd told stories of the war, his time in Hawaii logging shipments of supplies, his nickname—"Pay," short for Paymaster. He'd pointed out to me how, in civilian life, he continued in many Navy procedures, such as checking off items on his grocery store receipt and initial grocery list against the items he'd actually bought.

In my desk drawer, I keep two portraits of him in uniform, safe in the small light-brown leather folder Mom took with her to Montreal during the war. Every time I open that drawer, I see them and remember those khaki slacks.

X.

In 2006, he looked along the beach toward the path around the point, then back to me. "Can we walk out there?"

"If you like." I tried to quash my nerves. He'd managed it a few times this summer.

The sandy strip of beach gave way to stones covered with pine needles and dead leaves, creating a winding, uphill route through the woods. I stayed close behind him, wary of his leather shoes on pine needles—with reason, as it turned out. His soles slipped a bit and he wobbled.

Of their own accord, my hands found his slight upper body and braced him into balance. They stayed on his upper arms until the path was flat again. He nodded his thanks.

The path twisted between giant rocks left behind as glaciers retreated. He reached out to rap his knuckles against one.

He pushed it—a boulder the size of a small car or a baby elephant. Then he leaned his full weight, all 120 pounds, against it. He cast a sideways glance to be sure I'm watching.

"Sisyphean." I offered the smile he sought.

He lifted his hand to acknowledge my contribution before resuming careful steps along the path. On this sight-seeing trip, every stop held a memory.

At the end of the path, he hooked his thumbs into the waistband of his pants and looked up. He took a deep breath, so I did, too. I noticed the moist, cool air, the many soft shades of green around me. Water.

XI.

After my mother died, my father turned to his community. He joined the church choir. He went to steak dinners at the American Legion with fellow veterans. He met with the League of Women Voters, who asked for help making sense of the Electoral College after George W. Bush was elected in 2000.

Some things didn't change. He never could throw away rubber bands or fast-food condiment packets. He couldn't toss out any of the papers on which he'd written down his twice-daily blood pressure numbers. He kept a frustrating amount of *stuff*—church bulletins cascading from piles in his study, musty magazines stacked on shelves in the basement, empty cardboard boxes tucked under the stairs.

But he travelled—not easy for a man then in his eighties—to spend holidays with the five of us and our families, and to the lake. He talked to us regularly on the phone. He learned to say, "I love you."

Or perhaps I simply learned to hear it. To read him.

XII.

Dad and I began the return trip to the beach. I hovered behind him, my hands a bare inch behind his elbows but out of his range of vision, ready to support at the smallest hint of instability.

But he reached the beach without mishap. He paused to check the distance to the beach chairs, and trundled with careful steps over the shifting rocky sand, fists clenched with the effort. I drifted from behind him to his side so he could see that I trusted his tenacity.

At the chairs, he sat, his breaths open-mouthed and husky. We lingered, pretending we sat to enjoy the scenery a while longer. He closed his eyes and I watched his arms relax, his hands open. After about ten breaths, he closed his mouth and breathed through his nose again. About five more deep breaths, and he opened his eyes.

His breathing had eased but hadn't yet become something to take for granted.

He pointed to the gull. "Our friend is here."

The gull rolled and dove before resuming its watchful waiting. As we sat, it dove again, fruitlessly.

"He's not very good at fishing." Dad's voice held something. Wistfulness? Regret?

"Perhaps he has other talents."

"Perhaps."

And then my father began to talk. He stared out over the water, but I watched him, listening intently so I could hear him over the waves.

He described the summers he came to camp with my mother, starting in 1945, when he was back from Hawaii in time for V-E Day. One summer included side trips researching his Ph.D. dissertation, which he'd abandoned in 1942 to enlist in the Navy. In 1947, he and my mother didn't make the long drive from the East Coast of the U.S. to the lake because they were expecting their first child, the baby that died the following January.

He meandered through stories inspired by stories layered upon stories that branched into stories and returned to summers.

The gull hovered above us.

At last, he reached 1950 and the birth of my oldest brother. He checked his watch.

"Well." He stood up. It was time.

I don't remember all the stories he told that morning, and I don't think he expected me to. I think he just wanted to tell them again in that place, in the presence of those rocks and balsams and birch. And the gull. And the water.

XIII.

Like water, time appears in different ways in different landscapes. At home, photos show slabs of basalt along the lakeshore in the same places they were almost a century ago, when my mother waded there as a little girl. The trees have grown and changed. Alder thickets flourish, overgrow, thin, and flourish again. Cedars grow more slowly—a ten-year-old cedar might reach a height of three feet.

Meanwhile, a ten-year-old saguaro cactus is one inch tall. Sixty years later, at about six feet tall, it starts generating white flowers in the spring and red fruit in the summer. By the time it produces its first arm, at about fifteen feet tall, it can be 100 years old, a decade older than my father was during what turned out to be his last illness.

XIV.

In 2007, after a few days in the Coronary ICU, my father woke from sedation and was weaned from the ventilator. To gauge his mental acuity, the staff asked him who the president was.

"George W. Bush, but only for another year, nine months, and some-odd days." He couldn't repress a sigh, though he also smiled.

He recuperated enough to transfer to a rehabilitation centre to rebuild his strength. Roy joined me in Tucson and we spent every day with my father. Between my father's occupational and physical therapy sessions, we chatted, read, or sat in the sun in companionable silence. Sue came in after her work day, bringing entertainment—magazines, mail, news. One Sunday, we coloured Easter eggs.

But after a couple of weeks, my father's progress plateaued. He could never quite defeat the lung infection, and his body began to shut down. He returned to the hospital and asked to be admitted to hospice care. Once comfortable there, he sent Sue and Roy and me home to sleep. As the night became morning, he allowed his spirit to float away.

On that April Sunday morning, Sue and I sat with his body in the hospice room, where birds chittered at the feeder outside the window and cacti of all types watched from a respectful distance. She and I talked and were silent; we cried and laughed.

And in the hour we spent with my father, readying ourselves for whatever happened next, the white bristle of beard grew pronounced on his cheeks.

13

FIGHT FLIGHT FREEZE

It's early March when I finally challenge my fear of winter.

Even after several years of living year-round in Northwestern Ontario, I find winter daunting. The other new-to-me seasons intimidate me less. Spring is short—frantic and joyous. Autumn is all colour and crispness. But winter lies heavy on the land near the lake. Its painful cold and bitter winds arrive early and linger late into the year. Winter holds very real dangers.

It's time to embrace winter—to become as familiar with it as I am with the other seasons. I've made progress, but I'm still afraid.

Fear and I are old friends; it's my daily travelling companion. I'm afraid of lots of things: of dying, naturally, and of failure—sometimes I'm even afraid of trying. And, perversely, I'm also afraid of *not* trying, *not* living. Most of the time, however, fear of *not* doing something is less troublesome. *Not* climbing a mountain, supported only by rubber bands and metal? That's okay with me.

However, sometimes I want to try something, only to run up against the limits of my courage. More than once I have climbed back down the ladder of the three-metre diving board, unable to step into thin air, though it seemed possible from the ground. The teasing of my friends, however humiliating, was easier to endure than plummeting through empty space.

From what I've read, fear is both a basic part of life and physiologically complicated. Neurologists disagree about the validity of assigning unique functions to specific brain areas. Still, in recent research, the big players in the brain's fear response remain the amygdalae, the prefrontal cortex, and the hippocampus.

Our amygdalae are highly sensitive areas, and there's one in each brain hemisphere. They monitor everything happening around us. When presented with something that might be threatening, the amygdalae alert our prefrontal cortex, the part of the brain that decides whether to respond to the alarm or ignore it. In making its decision, the prefrontal cortex considers information from the hippocampus, which holds memories of related events. Over time, the whole system learns what is and isn't an actual threat to safety.

To become comfortable in winter, I've started teaching my brain about it. As a first step, I've started cross-country skiing. However, skiing isn't natural to me.

At the most trivial level, I can't figure out what to wear. I dress in layers, as everyone suggests, but that means I start frigid and stiff-limbed and become red-faced with fogged glasses after a few minutes. The equipment itself feels unwieldy. While clipping my boots to the skis, I mash my toe clip into the bindings without success, then try again while pushing at buttons with the tip of a pole and balancing (maybe) on the other foot. Whatever way I hold the poles feels awkward. Then the actual skiing brings its own terrors. The path that curves gently around small hills in summer transforms, with snow, into a series of apparently treacherous switchbacks and steep drops.

Roy has coached and encouraged me. In spite of my tense clumsiness, I have gained confidence in the gentle kick and glide, the shifts of balance necessary to take slow turns and small hills. Finally, I have learned to relax. A little.

That March Saturday, Roy asks if I want to ski on the lake ice. He means it. He's inviting me to ski on ice over water that remains extremely cold in summer, water that can freeze you senseless in minutes during the rest of the year. He and I have talked before, in passing, of skiing on the ice. When we were indoors and sipping coffee. When *yes* meant *someday*, and *someday* wasn't *now*.

It had all seemed so possible, when I sat in the chair by the fire. "Sure," I'd said. But now, as I think of the lake ice, I can practically feel my amygdalae thrumming.

We gear up and ski along the curving path to the camp. My assurance grows with each successful stride. *Maybe I can do this*, I think, but I don't tempt Fate by saying it aloud. We head around the camp to the lakeshore. I pause where, in the summer, the rocky beach becomes water, a transition point now covered in snow.

Roy leads the way onto the lake ice, here invisible under two inches of snow. I don't move. If it were possible, I would wring my mittened hands. As it is, I think *snow on ice, ice over water—deathly cold water*.

Neurologists say that in response to perceived threats, mammals have three innate options: to fight, to flee, or to freeze. I rarely fight. Fleeing is my go-to choice. Sometimes I freeze, though not in the sense that neurologists mean, an extreme state of shutdown—loss of consciousness, "leaving your body," that kind of thing. When I say "freeze," I mean only that I try not to run away until I get my bearings and choose a response instead of simply reacting.

This time, I succeed. After several deep breaths, I follow Roy. The reward comes immediately. Near the shore, skiing on the ice proves magical. I glide along the curving beach, so familiar in summer yet now bound by winter. Here, I feel comfortable. For one thing, the ice is camouflaged by several inches of snow; I could be skiing over a grassy field. For another, the water under the ice, when it *is* water, is shallow—maybe eight inches deep. I wonder what was so frightening a few moments ago; what could possibly scare me about this enchanting experience?

I approach the rocky spit of land that marks the outside edge of my family's secluded summer world. Around this point lies a larger bay, dotted with camps and newer, larger homes. As I near the tip of the point, I stop to look around. Behind and to the left, our yellow camp sleeps, tucked into the snow, with birch and balsams standing guard. To the right, the ice stretches, unbroken, to the familiar islands miles away. I look down between my ski tips at the ice peeking through the covering snow. It's clear, needled in white, over dark green water, and I remember that the water here is at least ten feet deep. I don't know how thick the ice is that protects me from the water. I don't even know how to gauge it.

I stand at the edge of a patch of bare ice, ten yards across, and as wide as I can see. No way around it. I will have to ski over it. And all my fears resurface. Maybe ice only pretends to be a solid. What if it remains water at its soul? How can I trust it with my weight?

Logic tries to coax me across. Before venturing out, I've researched "safety" and "lake ice." Many generations of many different peoples have lived with ice and skied on it. Inuit, Inupiat, Yupik; Swedes and Finns and Swede-Finns. All of them find ice sturdy and dependable in winter. In their worlds, ice roads are lifelines; they support transport trucks loaded with food and fuel. Governments even have regulations: according to the Minnesota Department of Natural Resources, clear blue ice that's roughly four inches thick is deemed safe for ice fishing; eight to twelve inches can support a car or small pickup truck.

I don't need an ice auger and ruler to know that this ice is safe. I have only to look: Roy waits on the other side of this ice patch.

Still, this is all just facts and logic—none of it makes any difference to my sweating palms, my immobile ski tips. To my amygdalae.

So I stand still. On skis. On ice.

In the Oklahoma of my childhood, snow came only rarely. We were more familiar with its cousin, black ice, which appeared in savage slicks on our winter roads. Ice in the forecast inspired dread. We tried to prepare for it, mentally, when it was only a distant threat. A "good winter" brought daytime temperatures in the forties Fahrenheit, with lows dipping to twenty—and no ice.

Even in Thunder Bay, where winter brings more snow than ice and ploughing works wonders on the streets, staying upright on sidewalks can be tricky during freeze-thaw-freeze cycles. A fall can break the spirit as well as the bones.

As I stand on skis on ice, I wonder—if I fall on the clear, needled ice, will it break underneath me? It seems both a certainty and a ridiculous impossibility. But I don't know enough about ice to know which is true.

I stall for time, and the sounds of winter surprise me again. Postcards of winter show scenes hushed by snow. But skiing isn't quiet. My poles crunch hard bites from snow; the skis hiss in turns. When I pause, bird sounds surface. Sparrows twitter at chickadees. Crows taunt each other like adolescent boys.

That Saturday, I also hear the ice. Sometimes it sounds like a slamming car door. Other times, it's a muffled torpedo launch, a bleating whale, a door creak, a dog in a sleepy, groaning stretch. All rough sounds, like complaints. On calm summer days, the lake breathes near-silent sighs and murmurs. But the lake's winter breathing is loud and requires more effort. The lake must get tired. When will she abandon the work of staying solid and become the water I know? The day is warm for early March; will *someday* become *now*?

Standing in the sun on this slick surface, miracles and catastrophes seem equally possible. So far, skiing on the ice has felt miraculous. But what's next?

I hear a long, reverberating crack. A gunshot? Is the ice breaking up? Does this sound mean catastrophe? My muscles tense; my ears ring. I hold my breath.

"That's just the ice settling," Roy says from the other side of the bare patch. "It's still safe."

I want to believe him. My prefrontal cortex is not so sure. My amygdalae are positive he's wrong; they're sounding every alarm they have.

Catastrophe marks time into "before" and "after."

The morning my father-in-law died unexpectedly, the sunlight seemed suddenly different. I saw strangers shopping for groceries, untouched by my catastrophe, and I wanted to shout into their faces, Don't you know he's gone?

And late in the disease that had taken from her whole vocabularies, homes, and lifetimes, my mother called me by name. I had thought her long gone, too far from shore to speak to me anymore, but she looked at me and said my name. In that moment, I inhaled in a different world.

But with time, "before" can blur into "after." Bad or good, moments are just that—moments. Another breath comes just after. Inhale, exhale.

People buy food in grocery stores and talk with their families, they strap on skis and venture onto ice. Disregarding weather puts them in harm's way. Or they're simply in the wrong place at the wrong time. They're lucky, they're grateful, they feel foolish, they learn lessons—or they don't. People die, and others sit in churches and mourn, and then they leave. They go to work or school the next day, and the next. Moments, like distances, accumulate.

After the shock of the cracking ice, I stand in a crevasse of "between." Behind me lies safety. I can go back along the shallow bit of shore to the land and wait for summer, as I have backed down the high dive, as I have so often failed in the face of my fears. This icy afternoon could be just another of those adventures that only *seem* possible. I can, I tell myself, try again another *someday*.

But.

I want to let this ice-world touch me. I want *someday* to become *today*.

Ignoring the alarms tingling in my palms, I take a breath and push backward with one foot. A tap and an out-of-control, quickly slowing slide. Unbeautiful and without grace, I nevertheless stay upright. Another tap, a slipping slide. Another, and another.

Finally, momentum carries me across the last of the bare ice and deposits me, upright, on the snowy surface beyond. Safe.

I exhale, and breathe again. My hippocampus has a new memory to integrate, one in which I skied across ice without catastrophe. My prefrontal cortex will consider it the next time I ski, and there will be a next time.

That winter and for winters to come, I will continue to accumulate experiences and memories, even though I'll remain a cautious person, respectful of the lake, winter as well as summer.

Roy and I ski home.

14

BIG IDEAS, SMALL FEET

"Not a creature was stirring...." (Clement Clarke Moore)

It was a typical summer night by the lake. The July twilight lingered past 11:00. My sister and I fell asleep as the sky deepened to navy blue, dotted with stars, for a few hours. Between 5:00 and 6:00 a.m., a soft grey replaced the darkness.

As I surfaced from sleep, I heard an odd rustling. More like a tapping. I tried to identify it: not a branch at the window; not a squirrel on the roof. No, the sound came from inside our small camp. Drowsy in my rumpled bedding on a cot in front of the row of windows facing Lake Superior, I put on my glasses and raised my head.

Not twenty feet away, in the kitchen, I saw it: a mouse, at eye level, on the counter, scurrying between boxes of crackers and a tin of cocoa.

I clutched the sheet to my chest and sat up, only to see something worse. Not mouse: mice. Plural.

I hate mice, but I don't just hate them: I loathe them, I'm revolted by them. Mice in the house, in the kitchen, *while I slept*: terrifying. Is it any wonder that I shrieked?

I'm not usually squeamish. Roy and I live on ten rural, forested acres along Lake Superior. We're casual about dirt and bugs, though I do appreciate the comforts of warm showers and insect repellant.

But in the years since I moved here, I've been sorting out complicated feelings. Somehow, I hadn't recognized that I'd be living in the country, not a small town. My transition from summer visitor to full-time owner didn't proceed along an orderly, linear path. The daily decisions we face continue to challenge me.

Consider the trees around our home. With all the talk of planting trees to offset carbon use, it's hard not to feel guilty about cutting trees down or even pruning branches. Yet we don't want trees to fall on our home, and we like to look at the lake. Are those good enough reasons to take them out?

Reading Robin Wall Kimmerer's 2013 book, *Braiding Sweetgrass*, reassured me. She writes about language, ceremony, and restoration, as well as the stories we tell ourselves about how to live. She encourages us to consider ourselves part of the planet's natural system. We're not entitled to abuse the world around us, but we can't help leaving our mark. And each place is unique, as we are—successful rewarding relationships don't look the same from person to person and place to place.

Inspired by her work, I decided to get to know our acreage. I'd watch and learn and try to adapt to its rhythms before bending it to my own preferences. Perhaps, eventually I could become a good steward of this land I love so much.

"The best-laid plans...." (Robert Burns)

That July morning, Sue, my sister, sleeping soundly in the cot just beyond mine, woke to my ear-ringing shriek, anguished and raucous. She started upright to see me crouched on all fours on my air mattress.

"What's *wrong*?" she demanded.

My response? Apparently, an agonized cry: "Miiiiice. T-TWO of them!"

I don't actually remember those moments. For me, they exist as feelings: disgust, horror, repugnance, slightly different but intense shades of hatred and fear. Everything else for me—even, to a certain extent, consciousness—had disappeared completely.

All those hopes for "getting to know the place" disappeared with the *skritch-skritch* scurrying of those little feet.

That year, as in most summers since our parents died, I had cleared the responsibilities from my regular life to vacation when my sister visited. For two weeks, we stayed in the small camp without electric power, though we heated our morning coffee on a propane cookstove. For entertainment, we went out in the rowboat, sat on the beach, monitored the growth of duck families, watched for loons, played in the water, and generally goofed off. We enjoyed some amenities—we showered at the house where I live with Roy the rest of the year, and we joined Roy there for most evening meals.

I often found it difficult to relax at camp. For years, we'd had just the time of our vacation to maintain two places. I kept seeing things I wanted to change—rooms to paint, paths to re-clear, grass to cut. Even with fifty other weeks in the year for chores, I couldn't always stop for those two.

I'd tried to cope by cultivating the gaze of my childhood, when imperfections were simply part of the package of play and adventure. Most summers, I regressed successfully enough to enjoy Sue's visit. Although every summer was different, every summer included the same elements: the camp structure, waterfowl, the birches, the lake, the rowboat.

And, that summer, a few mice.

Those mice forced me to view the camps in yet another way. I couldn't be a child and ignore the intruders. Yet I wanted to do something beyond reacting with disgust. How would a long-term steward respond to the problem of mice in the house? Probably not by screaming.

> *"...the world will beat a path to your door."*
> *(a misquote of Ralph Waldo Emerson)*

I don't know why mice affect me so. I'm mostly okay with ants (Sue's special fear). Keeping up with spiders and cobwebs in this region is difficult, but I can do it without flinching.

And perhaps there is no "why" to my loathing of mice. Perhaps it's my lizard brain at work, my highly developed sense of primal fear on overdrive.

I tried logic. Mice carry disease, but I can take precautions so that I don't endanger my health or that of my family, even at camp. As long as I don't step on one, I won't be bitten. If I keep the house free of accessible food, I likely won't see them, though they still may come in for shelter.

Unseen mice? Not reassuring.

The most effective course of action would be to keep them out of the camp. Experts recommend wedging steel wool into all holes and cracks in the foundation and plugging the surprisingly small crevices between floors and walls through which a mouse can squeeze. We can close doors.

But, as I continually reminded myself, fear isn't logical. Whatever success I'd had in retraining my brain to see skiing on ice as fun didn't transfer to mice at camp.

That summer morning, the best I could do was control the nausea. "Not puking" felt like a huge victory. Refraining from further shrieking took all the courage I could muster.

Fortunately, Sue is older and used to taking charge. She responded with the only weapons she had: sound and light. She shouted (profanity, I have to say) at the mice and trained a flashlight on them. Much later, when I ungratefully laughed at her efforts, she responded, reasonably, that she thought small nocturnal woodland creatures would be afraid of bright light and loud noises.

Perhaps they were: they certainly ran. One headed toward the back kitchen. The other ran TOWARD ME into the main room, where I still kneeled on my cot, as far away as possible from anything I thought mice could climb. As Sue opened the kitchen door and chased one into the back kitchen, I tried, through nausea, to keep tabs on the other. It kept disappearing, but I couldn't see where it went.

Finally we realized that the mouse was hiding behind the rocking chair's rockers, not scampering along the baseboard. Sue chased it into the kitchen, too, where it disappeared behind the wood cookstove. Neither of us could see it, nor a place where it could have escaped. Apparently, mice have a portal to an alternate universe. We gave up the chase.

"What now?" Sue asked, as she came back into the main room.

"Mousetraps." I took another deep, cleansing breath. "In the back kitchen." Where at least one mouse had scurried.

"What for bait?"

"Peanut butter."

"Are you comfortable setting traps?" Fair question on her part, since I was still on my cot.

"No, but I'm comfortable asking Roy to."

My mother would have rolled her eyes at my squeamishness. She had little patience with extremes of emotion. One of her biggest insults was to call someone "dramatic." She'd have urged me to grow up, get over it, and set my own mousetraps.

However, I knew that Roy excelled at handling things like mousetraps. So with my mother's endless lectures on self-reliance and independence echoing in my ears, I walked over to the house to ask for help.

Along the way, I enumerated all the ways in which I'd failed. I hadn't adequately prepared for two weeks at camp. I didn't have my rubber boots or any proper closed-toe shoes—the weather had been too warm to think of wearing them. I didn't even have long pants or socks.

At the house, I retrieved all those things, while Roy, laughing, went for the peanut butter.

Back at the camp, he asked where we'd seen the mice and where they'd disappeared to. He set two traps in the back kitchen and two in the kitchen proper. After cheerfully predicting that we wouldn't see them again until twilight, he left Sue and me to our vacation.

Adrenalin kept me buzzing, just putting in time until the mice came back. At least I had some armour: knee-high rubber boots especially helped me feel less vulnerable.

Eventually, Sue lured me down to the beach for breakfast. We went out in the rowboat. We played with art supplies, painting various types of leaves and ferns with student-grade acrylics and printing impressions on index cards.

I returned to my vow to experience the place without judgment. I noticed a few things: How the beach differed this year from lower-water years. How the grasses and small cedars at the edge of the rocky shoreline continued to thrive, even with their roots underwater. How lighting a fire in the wood stove, even on a rare warm-ish morning in the misty, damp summer, helped dry the air and made our place feel cozy and safe again.

Safe for us humans, that is.

"A mouse does not rely on just one hole." (Plautus)

Over our sketchbooks, Sue and I also talked about the ethics of mousetraps and mousetrap placement. She wondered if the two traps in the back kitchen, which we don't even try to secure fully against the outdoors, might lure in mice that would otherwise have stayed outside. (I suspect she also wondered if setting four traps inside the main camp structure would capture more intruders, but she was kind enough not to plant this idea in my head.)

We talked briefly about other methods of keeping them out. I was completely uninterested in live traps. I wanted to ensure that the mice, once inside and caught, would never have the opportunity to come *back* inside.

On the other hand, poison seemed like an overreaction. We didn't want to kill all mice everywhere (though I did fantasize about that, briefly), only the ones that crossed the barriers that marked "indoors." I was okay (almost) with mice living in the entire rest of the world, if they stayed out of this camp while I was there.

That evening, as we sat watching light linger on the lake, Sue and I heard two snaps from the back kitchen. Although I tried to be brave and pick up mouse-and-trap for disposal, even donning a large plasticized glove, I couldn't override my instinct to stay far away. Again, Sue had to be the brave big sister and deal with reality.

Two more snaps during the night helped transform my disgust to annoyance. Those mice didn't care at all about my feelings. Couldn't they give me even 800 square feet of mouse-free space?

No. They could not.

> *"The early bird may get the worm,*
> *but it's the second mouse that gets the cheese"*
> *(Ernest Berg)*

I'm embarrassed to have responded to the mice so...what's the word? Viscerally? Cravenly? But I try to remember that relationships develop over time, as you work with what *is* true instead of what you *wish* were true. Allowing for give-and-take is part of the package.

Roy and I will always prune branches that encroach onto walking paths. We'll need to keep an eye on the alder and Manitoba maple so they don't crowd out everything else. Every year, we'll have deadfall to manage and firewood to stack. We'll never be "done" with projects, any more than the trees are ever "done" with their cycle of growing leaves, shedding them, and growing them again in the ongoing march of seasons.

But. Some realities are easier to accept than others.

I'm unhappy that our battle against mice may never be over. That summer, after two nights of full traps, Roy and I plugged holes in the camp foundation, and our rate of capture slowed. By the end of Sue's visit, our grand total was thirteen.

When I resumed my regular life at the house, we left behind baited traps at camp. I checked them throughout the rest of the summer and, finding nothing, I allowed myself to hope we'd eradicated their ingress points. However, when the weather turned cooler again in late September, we had three more. We'll need to check the floor under the piano again—a project for another summer.

Sue is probably looking forward to a summer with nights uninterrupted by shrieks, snaps, or both. She gave me one of my best laughs of the summer when she dug into the peanut butter with a spoon, saying, "Why should the mice have *all* the fun?"

But I can't expect her to do the hard work. I need and want to learn new skills.

And, fortunately or not, I'll have that opportunity. My office is in the basement of the house, and recently I saw a mouse streak across the floor into the one inaccessible corner, behind the filing cabinet. (Yes, I shrieked, but only once!) Although this mouse and its friends have so far ignored the freshly set, peanut butter–laden mousetraps, I know it's only a matter of time before I hear their scurrying feet.

15

DRIFTGLASS

Today, Lake Superior in our little cove lies mostly flat, with just a few breaths to ruffle the water's surface. On this calm, late-spring day, it's hard to picture the winter storms whose pounding surf changes the contents and shape of this beach.

As always when I walk, I have two pockets, right and left, sheep and goats, treasures and trash. I don't actually walk, though, as much as I meander, bending and straightening, looking for what's out of place, what's been left, what's not right.

***

On the beach, I don't court memories. I don't have to. Simply creating space—a quiet hour's solitude one afternoon on our sand-and-rock beach—gives them permission to appear.

I bend over to pick up something that catches my eye. It's hard with an irregular shape, mostly flat, about the size of a quarter, pinkish-purplish and made opaque by sand. As I turn it over in my palm, admiring the colour, I'm a young adult again, in a department store with my mother. We pass between rows of sheets and towels, and she slows and touches my arm.

"What do you think of these?"

Intent on other errands, I glance where she points. A set of tan bedsheets features a scissor-tailed bird of paradise, black-and-white head, blue and fuchsia feathers, sitting on a branch and surrounded by white lush flowers crimped in pink and rose and lilac.

"Eh. Looks like something you'd like. Not really my preference."

Years later, I wince, hearing again the shrug in my voice and registering, too late, the over-elaborate casualness of her question.

And I hear again her response. "Ah. Uh-huh." And, across her face, a flash of something—sadness? Disappointment?

A few days after that shopping trip, my family gathers for dinner to celebrate my graduation, and I open gifts. Among them, that set of sheets, purchased before she asked my opinion in the store. I thank my mother, and my gratitude is sincere—sheets are expensive on a budget as small as mine, and I'm happy to use whatever sheets I get.

But her eyes hold sadness, and her rueful smile is an apology. What for? For not correctly guessing my taste? For not knowing me as well as she thought?

Some thirty-five years later, I still feel sad.

* * *

On a beach walk, I look at colours.

Underwater, stones sparkle. Sandstones gleam in bright persimmon and ground ginger.

On the beach, the sandstones' colours are softer, dustier cinnamon sticks and caramels among the dull greys and charcoals of the granites and basalts.

Once my eyes become accustomed to the palette, I readily notice other colours. Colours of mistakes, of objects tossed and lost, discarded or forgotten.

* * *

For years, I've wondered why I didn't clue in to what my mother really needed that afternoon in the department store.

In retrospect, I see that she was setting up a later moment, one we'd share. In her version, as I opened gifts at that family party, our eyes would meet across the room. She wouldn't need to say, "Remember seeing those in the store? I just loved them and I knew you would, too." That shared glance of perfect understanding would be enough to reinforce our mother-daughter bond.

Even at the time, I heard something in her voice—wistfulness, a need for connection, reassurance that although I was embarking on a life of my own, she still knew me. That although her youngest child was leaving home, she still had something to offer.

It all felt like a test, one I'd failed.

A counsellor told me I'd done nothing wrong. My mother had asked a simple question, and I'd answered honestly. Furthermore, I had difficulty making decisions, big and small—with five kids, my mother kept order by limiting the number of choices we could make. As the youngest, I had few options to begin with, and most were second-guessed by older family members. Long into adulthood, selecting bedding for a new apartment was as stressful to me as finding the apartment itself.

But that perspective, and my counsellor's absolution, don't keep me from turning over that memory. Worrying it. Holding it up to the light like my piece of driftglass, watching the pinks shift and sparkle. Setting it down, only to pick it up again.

*　*　*

My grandparents loved photography. Family albums include shots of my mother as a girl in a middy blouse, mugging for the camera. My uncle poles unstable-looking rafts.

My mother and uncle and aunt, in church clothes, pose for my grandmother. A collared shirt and tie can't make my uncle's spiky hair look respectable. My mother, all of twelve, peers out from her cloche. My three-year-old aunt's white stockings sag at the knee. They lean on a giant chunk of basalt, where several decades of August days later, my siblings and I ate sandwiches and soup and Ontario peaches.

I've seen those photos so often that the images become part of my memories.

My sister and my aunt as swimsuited teenagers, in pictures taken twenty-five years apart, adopt similar poses—one hand on an outthrust hip, the other behind the head, elbow high.

My four older siblings as young children sit on the raft, its pole twice as tall as any of them.

I also remember generalities, the "things that always happened." A keening gull, a raven's inquisitive cackle. Murmured grunts from mother ducks escorting a flotilla of ducklings out of danger. Canoe paddles dipping and dripping. The squeal of the rowboat's oarlocks. In my palm, a smooth dark rock for skipping, its top sun-warm, its sandy bottom cool.

When I wander the beach long enough, flashes of my own specific memories surface.

I'm younger, in high school. The summer morning sun warms the sand underfoot. My mother stands bent over in front of me, scrubbing shampoo from her hair as I slosh cold water over her head. I lift the metal bucket high, aiming at the crown of her head, but the water lands on the nape of her neck.

Both of us are laughing.

"Ooof! Brrr."

"Sorry."

We laugh because we knew it would be like this—the shock of the icy water, stray runnels flowing down and around her neck to drip onto the beach despite my careful aim. I didn't splash her purposely; her discomfort was not my fault.

That day, we both knew it.

* * *

So many colours and memories.

Blue on the lake horizon, in the sky—acceptable, unremarkable. Blue on the beach—often a plastic bottle cap. I'm sure it wasn't there yesterday, or last week, or the last time I was here.

White gulls overhead, white boats, white birch trunks—all appropriate on this late-spring afternoon. White on the beach—sometimes curls of birchbark, sometimes a quartz nugget, but often plastic labels, sandwich bags, or the brittle-thin plastic of a broken fishing float.

And sometimes the white is a bit of glass, originally clear but scoured white by sand. Our family knows it as driftglass; others call it beach glass or sea glass.

We also find pieces that are cobalt blue, light and dark green, brown. Older pieces of clear glass—like the one I spotted this late-spring day—contain additives that turn shades of pink and lavender in decades of sunlight.

Pieces of plastic and other garbage go into my left pocket, driftglass into my right. Goats and sheep. Trash and treasures, mistakes the genesis of both.

* * *

I can't stop thinking about those sheets and my mother that day. I feel ridiculous, spending so much time thinking about mundane objects. But I can't seem to let it go. I wonder why she set herself up—and me, too—for embarrassment and disappointment.

Or perhaps it was a show of confidence. Years earlier, she'd trusted me with that bucket of cold water. Was she equally sure I'd know the right thing to say about the sheets?

Did my blunder—my failure to understand her need to connect—change how she felt about me? Or did that incident fade, becoming just one of many stones on her beach?

Maybe it was a test, and *she* felt she'd failed somehow.

I used those sheets for years without really thinking about whether I liked them. In my thirties, I realized how much I loved them, and not only because I was used to seeing them. The bird had become striking and exquisite to me, the flowers exuberant. I grew into those sheets. My mother had been right. Only her timing had been wrong.

I turn the piece of glass over and over, rubbing it between my fingers. Later, I'll add it to the pile of driftglass in the silver bowl in the dining room.

I doubt I'm finished with that memory—it'll probably surface on another beach walk. If not that specific memory, another one. I'll be making sense of my relationship with my mother for some time.

For now, the piece of pink driftglass goes into my right-hand pocket: a treasure.

16

ENTANGLEMENT

One recent morning, I went for a walk in the neighbourhood, paying attention to nothing other than the sweetness of the breeze on my face and the warm sun hugging my shoulders. And then I rounded a corner and saw him coming toward me—my dog, Sparky. And he saw me. And he grinned.

Joy flooded my body, as if my heart had never broken. My breath caught. He wanted to run to me, I just know he did, but he was on a leash.

He also wasn't Sparky. He stood at about the same height, his head just where I could rest my hand on it without stooping. He wore the same chestnut-and-black saddlebags on his fluffy white coat and walked with the same broad-chested prance. As always, his tail waved as if he led a parade up that street.

But he couldn't have been Sparky. I forced myself to breathe deeply.

As we passed, the dog laughed up at me, sharing the joy of being on a walk—*walking! going for a walk!*—on what had been a random Wednesday. I smiled at him and in the general direction of the person holding the leash, and I picked up my pace.

It's not Sparky, I reminded myself.

* * *

Then I ran a thought experiment—a flight of fancy followed to its natural conclusion. I find thought experiments beguiling. They're metaphors on steroids, elaborate games of "what if?" Using just your imagination, you can examine the very nature of the world. You can clarify an abstraction. You can illustrate a difficult idea.

Through the years, philosophers and scientists have used thought experiments to consider whether the universe has a boundary, how objects fall through space, and how gravity affects the orbits of moons and planets.

One of the most famous thought experiments involves a box holding not a dog, but a cat. In 1935, the Austrian physicist Erwin Schrödinger proposed an experiment to explore quantum events—specifically, how subatomic particles like photons and electrons interact. In his thought experiment, a cat is placed in a sealed box with a flask of poison, a source of radioactivity, a Geiger counter, and a hammer. If the Geiger counter detects any radioactive decay, it triggers the hammer, which shatters the flask of poison, which kills the cat. But if the radioactive material doesn't decay, the flask of poison remains intact, and the cat remains alive.

One way of thinking about quantum events, known as the Copenhagen interpretation, says that the cat in the box remains simultaneously both dead and alive until someone observes the outcome. Until then, all possible outcomes exist. A cat in the box remains both alive *and* dead; a photon is both a particle *and* a wave.

***

I first met Sparky when I started dating Mike. Sparky was already two years old by then, so I experienced his puppyhood through Mike's stories. Even though Sparky was the runt of a very mixed-breed litter, Mike had picked him because Sparky had scampered up to Mike with confidence. In truth, Sparky had picked Mike, right from the start.

Their early time together had its frustrations. As a young dog, Sparky loved to chew. One morning in early spring, a delivery service left a large box of CDs inside the gate to Mike's yard, and Sparky "opened" it. A snowstorm passed through that afternoon, leaving behind several inches of snow. Mike came home to a yard full of snow-covered lumps. A few CDs appeared when the snow finally melted the next week. For months, Mike found corrugated cardboard bits under bushes. The following summer, he unearthed a stray jewel box that had been partially buried in the flowerbed.

"Darn dog," Mike said, always with affection, at the end of the story. Because in spite of Sparky's chewing, he was impossible to resist: his cheerful white-furred face, with its one chestnut ear folded at a jaunty angle toward his hazel eyes, made up for a lot. He was easy to forgive, especially as he got older and channelled his energy into retrieving balls.

Though I'd missed Sparky's puppyhood, I had no trouble falling in love. Mike and I were also comfortably committed to each other. And Sparky liked having me around. Two humans doubled his chances that someone would throw something for him to bring back. He loved Fetch, using his upright, waving-flag tail to show his pride in being a *good boy, such a good boy*.

* * *

Schrödinger intended his cat-in-a-box thought experiment to show the shortcomings of the Copenhagen interpretation of quantum particle behaviour. He didn't think a photon could be both a particle and a wave. After all, a living-and-dead cat is impossible, according to how we experience the world.

But his thought experiment caught the public imagination, in spite of what he thought was its obvious absurdity. Those of us who aren't particle physicists, or even scientists, see near-miracles every day. We can peer inside our bodies and watch our hearts beat. Though half a world may separate family members, parents can read bedtime stories to their children, face-to-technology-to-face.

So someday, in this world of scientific advancements we don't fully understand, we might eventually have explanations of even the most complicated phenomena. Like love.

* * *

Mike never said, "Love me, love my dog," but the result was the same. Sparky was always part of our life together. But the relationships among the three of us weren't equal.

One long weekend soon after we started dating, we took a quick vacation in the mountains. Sparky panted over our shoulders from the back seat, curling up for a nap and then standing again to look out the window in the hope of spotting a deer to bark away.

We stopped for gas, and Mike went into the store to pay while I stayed in the car with Sparky. The moment Mike disappeared from his sight, Sparky began whining.

"It's okay, boy." I laid my hand on his head. "I'm still here."

Feet shifting in his Sit, he glanced at me—*who cares*, he all but said—and whimpered louder. I scratched behind his ears. He shook off my hand and stood up to check the windows—none open, no way to get out and find Mike. He sagged back into a disappointed, silent Sit. He looked at me.

"Good boy," I said. He sighed deep in his throat, ears on alert, except for the top of his left one, which folded down in its oh-so-adorable way. He as much as said, *Sure, he's always come back, but that was before. What if this time is different?*

But it wasn't different. And when Mike emerged from the convenience store, Sparky yelped with joy. I knew then that however much Sparky loved me—and he did, I was sure—Sparky was Mike's dog. To him, Mike came first.

I understood Sparky's devotion, I thought. Mike and I were compatible—he appreciated quippy humour and gentle teasing.

We both loved music and being outdoors. Mike came first in my life, and I came first in Mike's. That's how relationships work. You have each other's best interests at heart when you make decisions. Or so I thought.

* * *

It comforts me to know that scientists debate the nature of the particles, visible and invisible, that make up our world. I like knowing that they don't have all the answers, either. The world is a complex place, no matter how many ways we try to simplify it.

Sometimes, a group of subatomic particles interacts in a way that makes it impossible to determine the quantum state of the individual particles. Instead, you can describe the quantum state only of all of the particles together—the system as a whole. Schrödinger gave this form of interaction the German word *Verschränkung*, which he translated as *entanglement*.

* * *

Sparky, Mike, and me. Our life together felt so ... inevitable. Events followed, one upon another, and led to the expected outcome: we got married and had a puppy, Gizmo. Gizmo was pleasant enough to Mike and me but remained 100% Sparky's dog through the years.

The four of us played together, sledding and hiking. Sparky loved Fetch at the dog park, where he'd bring back the ball while Gizmo, a joyous runner, nipped at Sparky's heel and tail. Evenings, we'd cook with the dogs underfoot and then pile on the couch to watch TV. We made a family.

The earth turned on its axis and completed orbits around the sun. My aging parents lived 800 miles away—800 miles that felt like 800 light-years—and I made frequent trips to visit them. There, my father cared for my mother, whose Alzheimer's rapidly changed her personality and her abilities. I worried about them and tried to support them, but my nuclear family was back home, with Mike and "the boys."

Any time a suitcase appeared, Sparky whimpered and moped. He rallied quickly when I was the only one packing, but when Mike went on a business trip, Sparky spent much of the time resting his chin on the bedroom windowsill, waiting. Sometimes I'd sit next to him and lean against him. He'd lean back against me for a bit. Then, with a sigh, he'd bring me his ball for Fetch, for which he mustered about 85% enthusiasm.

I didn't take it personally. I missed Mike, too.

* * *

Einstein is said to have called entanglement "Spooky action at a distance." I amuse myself by thinking of it as "Sparky action at a distance."

In German, *Verschränkung* can also refer to the act of *folding together*. For example, as in the *clasping* of hands, perhaps across a table at a special anniversary celebration, or while two people walk through a sunny park together.

Also as in the *crossing* of your arms over your chest, perhaps while listening to a spouse's slurred explanation after a late arrival home, or while sitting in a marriage counsellor's office, apportioning blame.

* * *

Compare marriage to Schrödinger's cat-in-a-box experiment. Both are full of vulnerabilities. Glass flasks are fragile. So is life, cat or dog or human. Is a hammer inherently destructive? Maybe—it is, after all, an instrument of change. How about poison? It's lethal by definition, but only if someone chooses to make it so.

During one of those trips around the sun, Mike's father died unexpectedly of heart failure. My mother's death four months later was no less devastating for coming after long illness.

Both losses gave us new experiences of the world. In fact, they created new worlds, places we'd never lived before. They also exposed weaknesses that had underlain our marriage all along, undetected by our Geiger counters. At some point, Mike's jokes had grown sharp barbs. He stopped laughing with me, or even at me. Apparently, any time I had packed a suitcase, I'd chosen my parents over him. Or so he thought. Maybe. He became silent and stayed that way.

Although I've tried for years, I can't de-tangle the elements of the system that was our marriage. It doesn't really matter. Once the flask is destroyed, poison pervades the system. The outcome is what's important.

* * *

One necessary part of Schrödinger's thought experiment was a time limit—one hour, long enough that some radioactive decay *might* occur, but not so long that it *would*. Without a time limit, the cat would eventually die, one way or another. As do we all.

How long do you give someone—grieve someone—husband or dog? After years of trying to hold our family together, I had to accept just how many light years had come between Mike and me. In the version of the universe in which that marriage existed, I finally opened the box to see our marriage. Dead.

One late-August morning, I assembled cardboard boxes and began. For weeks, I sorted linens, knickknacks, music, artwork, and photos. While I worked, Gizmo crept under the bed and poked his nose out from under the dust ruffle, but Sparky sat near me. Occasionally, I'd toss his ball. By this time, Sparky was an old dog, almost fourteen, and although he was still devoted to Fetch, he could complete only a few trips before he needed a rest. Often, instead of chasing the ball, he'd simply sit and watch its arcing flight before turning back to me.

Eventually, it was time. My belongings—and one CD case with Sparky's teeth marks in it—sat packed in row of cardboard boxes. As I put the last lid on the last box, Sparky rested his chin on it for a moment before turning to lie down close beside me. He had whimpered when Mike and I raised our voices; he had listened, one ear alert and one drooping, during our ever-lengthening silences. He knew I would not be coming back.

They'll be fine *without me,* I told myself. Gizmo would still have Sparky, and Sparky would have Mike. I scratched behind Sparky's ears and dropped a kiss on the top of his dear, furry head.

* * *

Schrödinger's thought experiment wasn't the last theory scientists developed to explain quantum phenomena.

A newer one, the Many-Worlds theory, says that the act of observing the cat in the box doesn't irrevocably determine the outcome, either killing or sparing the cat. Instead, the universe creates a copy of itself for each possible outcome.

So according to the Many-Worlds theory, a universe exists in which the flask in the box is intact, and one in which it isn't—a universe, therefore, in which the cat lives, and one in which it dies.

* * *

More than a decade out of that marriage, I sometimes ask myself, "How could I have left him?"—but only about Sparky or Gizmo, never about Mike.

Still, I can do arithmetic. As much as I would love to believe that the dog I saw on my walk was Sparky, I also know it couldn't have been, based on the way we humans and dogs experience time.

But I cling to the Many-Worlds theory, and it helps mend my heart. I now think of Sparky in a parallel universe somewhere, where dogs live as long as our love for them does.

There, Sparky joyfully fetches a ball for someone he loves—maybe even for me.

(Names in this essay, though changed, remain entangled.)

17

NULLIPAROUS

ulliparous, 1959. Medical Latin. From *nulli-*, stem of *nullus*, "no" + *-para*, fem. of *parus*, from *parere* "to bring forth." Not + a woman brings forth. A woman who hasn't given birth.

* 0 *

Clickety clickety clack. My family physician peers at me from under her bangs, fingers still flying on her keyboard.

"Mother?"

"Dead." My voice is flat. "She was eighty-three. In 2000. Alzheimer's disease. Well, pneumonia, but you know."

I'm just there for a checkup. I'm never sick, beyond an annual cold. But I'm plenty sick of menopause—I can't seem to figure out how to do it right. And I haven't seen the doctor in so long that we're reviewing my family history.

I watch her. She's a few years older than I am, but probably not much over sixty. As she asks questions, she sometimes glances at me over her reading glasses but mostly looks at her laptop. I try not to feel judged.

She keeps typing as she starts her next question. "And, um, her…." Her voice trails off as she finishes her note without looking up. "Your mother's menopause. What was that like?"

"She had a hysterectomy in 1967, when she was, let's see, fifty. She'd had bleeding." I try to remember family stories while she types. "Fibroids, I think. They took her ovaries, too. She had estrogen shots afterwards, something like every six or eight weeks, until maybe 1980 or so. Maybe later."

I wish I'd paid attention to my mother's health earlier, for so many reasons that haven't stopped with her death. Like, when did she first notice her memory slipping—with menopause, or only later?

Clickety-clickety.

"How about your siblings, any sisters?"

"One. Nine years older. She had ovarian cancer in her early twenties."

Clack. The typing stops. "Oh."

That always gets attention. Meeting her eyes, I say, "But it's not that kind. Not related to BRCA. It's—I don't know the name. Contained? Though her ovary burst."

She shakes her head and resumes typing, and I wish I remembered the cancer type, but I babble on. "She had a hysterectomy, including ovaries. And radiation. She's fine now."

Clickety-clickety.

"Good. And that was…when?"

"Um…" I do arithmetic. "Forty years ago? Forty-five? Early seventies."

"No recurrence?"

Click clickity click.

I shake my head, adding "No" aloud as her eyes stay glued to the screen. I wait.

Click click. The typing stops.

"Hmm." She still doesn't look up. "So no natural menopause in your immediate family, then."

"Yes. Right. No." Not only am I not doing menopause right—my whole family hasn't, either.

* O *

* Perfect Devilled Eggs *

Eggs are difficult to cook properly. Science says so: the white and the yolk harden at different temperatures. And personal preference defines "properly" {runny yolk : runny white : both runny : both hard : something in between}. My first time, at ten or twelve, devilling eggs for Sunday dinner. My mother standing over me as I measure, timer and teaspoons; the need to "do it right" imprinted early. My sister still asks me to devil eggs when I visit her, or she visits me.

Devilled eggs are the only company-worthy dish I make. Decades of experience translate, in some small way, to skill. But I know, and science confirms, that eggs are difficult to cook properly, so I ask other women {only women: most men don't make devilled eggs} for their secrets. Everyone's secret is the opposite of someone else's.

* O *

Nulliparous: A medical term that, for me, is synonymous with "normal." Some medical conditions that sound ominous or pejorative simply describe a state of being. For example, if a medical condition has been defined that describes the state of "never having broken a bone," I also have that.

* O *

As my doctor points out, I'm going through menopause without help from family history. I have sussed out this fact myself. I ponder it in the night, when I kick sheets off my sweating body. When I am wakeful and cranky for no real reason.

Or rather, for many reasons I can and do enumerate in the dark, reasons that I recognize as the vicissitudes of daily life but that still feel monstrously, disproportionately unfair. Reasons such as not enough work, too much work. Rejected work, others' work chosen over mine. Plans for new writing that seem certain, in the night, to be rejected too.

Reasons that encompass the unsatisfactory nature of other areas of life. My marriage is fine; my husband is great, but there's always something. Household chores—laundry undone, refrigerator shelves in desperate need of purging, cupboard shelves half-empty, a roof that leaks when the rain comes on the northeast wind, a deck that needs shoring up.

Or, more personally, my hair, in all its permutations—what needs to be coloured or encouraged, what needs to be removed, and how, and how often. My other failings—my fluctuating weight, lack of physical fitness, incessantly itchy skin, iffy wardrobe, and overall lack of skill in navigating female adulthood.

Such as this particular rite of passage, menopause. In the night, I feel especially orphaned. If I think about it too much, I can make myself cry. Unless that's just sweat trickling down my face.

In the throes of hot-flashing insomnia, I flop from my back to my front and back again, punching and flipping my pillow as my husband snores undisturbed beside me. Finally, I give up and get up to pour a glass of water and read, trying not to think, *This is someone else's (unrejected) work.*

Of all the "gifts" of menopause, insomnia feels particularly cruel, creating as it does a theatre for pondering life's impermanences and impertinances. And sometimes along with all the rest that feels unfair, I ponder my family history, or rather, its lack. *How do we do menopause in our family?* I'll never know. I try to spin it to the positive: *I'll be the first! I'm blazing a trail! Literally!* Though I know "blazing" means something different when applied to a trail, I snort at my own joke and fan my face with my book.

Without any precedents, I've followed general advice for managing menopause. I have limited alcohol and sweets, exercised more, eaten more fruits and vegetables, and tried to keep regular hours for waking and sleeping. I can't find it in me to give up coffee, but I've cut my chocolate intake to one nightly bite.

Yet about half the nights, I lie frustrated and sweating, or get up to read, for several hours. Hence the doctor's appointment.

* O *

* Secrets for Boiling Eggs to Devil *

The eggs should be old, the ones that have been sitting in your refrigerator the longest. They should be fresh, from the farmer that day if you can get them.

Start with eggs that are room temperature. Get the eggs from the fridge into the pan quickly, while they're still cold as ice cubes.

Put them into a saucepan and run cold water—as cold as possible, just short of ice—from the tap until they're submerged. Cover them completely with hot tap water; you want to start them cooking right away.

Add a teaspoon of vinegar—that's the secret; it's absorbed through the shell. Vinegar in the cooking water does nothing beyond making the water smell.

Bring the water to a hard boil and boil the hell out of them for twenty minutes. Over medium heat, bring them to a gentle boil and turn down to simmer for about twelve minutes—no more, or that grey ring will form around the yolk.

* O *

Nulliparous: It's my default state. It's not so much that I *decided not to have children*. It's that I *never decided to have them*. My life's path has twisted and turned like anyone else's. I've arrived at intersections and made choices. I've even burned my fair share of bridges. But I didn't reach that particular crossroad until my hysterectomy.

* O *

Clickety-clack-clickety.
"Okay, now you. How long have you been in menopause?"
"Well, I don't know for sure. I haven't had a uterus since 1999." I keep my voice bland, though I'm a little alarmed at her question—isn't my chart right in front of her? I explain briefly.

A series of abnormal Pap smears. Two outpatient cone biopsies of my cervix over a three-year period, both negative for cancer. The last procedure, when I was thirty-eight, caused my cervix to heal closed. Hysterectomy was the only solution. I still have ovaries.

"Right."
Clicky-clickety.
"So, the other menopause symptoms, then. Hot flashes?"
"Yeah." I calculate. "Five years? Off and on?" I ignored them as long as I could.

She consults my date of birth—I'm fifty-five. "Only five years?" I hear a raised eyebrow in her voice.

I'm doing it wrong. "Maybe six? Not more, though."
Clickety-clickety.
"Okay. Back to your family; we'll just update all the sections of this form while we're at it. Pregnancies. How many times was your mother pregnant?"

"Um. At least seven that I know of. Their first baby died, and she had at least one miscarriage. And five of us."

"And your sister?"
Clickety-click.
I shake my head. "Hadn't had a chance."
"And you?"
Again, I shake my head. "No children. No pregnancies." My choice.

The glance from under the hair. "Hmmm."
Clickety click.

That choice. That's become a new concern for me in the wee hours. I was happily uninterested in having children for decades, but now my husband and I are making wills. Our physical assets can be divided and distributed to relatives, but what about the intangibles? Who will love this whole place—the ten acres my husband and I live on, part of which has been in my family since 1924—with the giddy reverence we do? Who will cherish the boxes in our basement, the ones holding a century's worth of my mother's family photographs and letters?

And one of my most selfish thoughts: who will be left to miss me?

I hear myself. I know that my insomnia is making it all about me, not acknowledging that the children I didn't have would have been their own joyous, independent, autonomous selves.

In the years in which I didn't have children, I didn't foresee these wakeful hours. Then again, I didn't foresee any part of menopause. I didn't know how it would feel—or that it would feel any way in particular. For me, menstruation had been a minor inconvenience at worst. I had no reason to imagine that menopause would be different.

But I hadn't seen it up close in a way I could remember or understand. I was six for my mother's surgery and eleven when my sister had cancer. When I was in high school, my mother mentioned lying awake at night, worrying about my four siblings, starting with the oldest and working her way down to me, but I hadn't connected her insomnia and worry to menopause or her estrogen shots.

Instead, I thought, "This is just *how she is*." A nighttime worrier. That's also what I thought in my mid-thirties, when "how she is" meant that Mom repeated stories, lost nouns, and felt mixed-up and confused. I clung to "how she is" until her diagnosis.

To be fair, our family didn't talk about difficult transitions of any type. Those stories were never told, not until I came along to write about my mother's Alzheimer's disease. Still, nothing about my mother's menopause is documented in those boxes in the basement.

Click clickety clickety.

I wonder what my physician keeps typing, since we've finished my family history. Eventually, she turns to me. "All right. We'll send you for several different tests."

I'm game. Whatever will help make me sleep better and feel less cranky.

She resumes typing. I watch the printer, where pieces of paper—orders for my tests—rise smoothly in the tray.

* 0 *

* Secrets for Peeling Eggs to Devil *

You have to shock them. Drain the saucepan and plunge the eggs in a bowl of ice water, then roll them around on the bottom of the bowl to crack the shell all over. Twist the shell slightly to break the membrane and slip the white out. Work fast.

Be gentle with them. Pour out some of the warm water. Then tilt the saucepan in the sink and run warm water over them, gradually changing to cooler and then finally cold. When the eggs are just cool enough to hold, leave a small stream of water running from the tap. Give the egg a smart rap against the sink, then hold the egg under the stream. The water will gentle off the shell and membrane.

It doesn't matter when you peel them—you can even leave them unpeeled in the fridge overnight if you want.

Really, too many variables are at play to claim that you know THE perfect method for peeling eggs.

* 0 *

Nulliparous: Physically, my hysterectomy was easy, but I'd be lying if I said it was easy to accept. I was angry.

It wasn't that I wanted to have kids after all.

It was partly that I'd been asking for a hysterectomy ever since my cervix showed abnormalities. If my cervix was only one or two steps away from cancer, I wanted it out. However, three different gynecologists, two of them male, had said I was too young, in my early thirties, to make that decision.

But mostly I was angry because until that surgery, having children had been *my* decision: I didn't have children. After the hysterectomy, I couldn't. That bridge lay in ashes behind me.

O

A few weeks after my checkup, I'm in my kitchen. A dozen eggs have bubbled and nudged each other in a saucepan. On the counter, I set a red bowl, part of the Corningware mixing-bowl set just like my mother's, and a red-handled paring knife that I took from her kitchen when we were emptying our family home. I fold a paper towel in half and set it beside the sink; I'll blot the eggs and wipe my knife blade on it. I pour steaming water from the pan into the sink and add cool tap water to cover them again.

Starting with my hand underwater, I crack the first egg. After I peel it, I cut it in half to be sure the yolk is solid. The white is too hot for me to handle much, but I manage to pop the yolk halves into the bowl. Then I start running a thin stream of water into the saucepan and, one by one, roll eggs against the stainless steel sink divider.

Crunchity-clickety-crunch.

The sound reminds me of my physician, first at her laptop and then brandishing the sheaf of orders for urine tests, blood tests, and a mammogram.

"This'll get us started," she says.

Her face, behind that mop of bangs. The first of many faces.

Two new faces at the lab. The dark eyes of the round-faced young male tech-in-training, skilled in blood draws but embarrassed to hand me the urinalysis cup. The amused indulgence in the smile of the woman, near my age, who coached him.

Another face. Two weeks after my doctor's appointment, the reassuring direct gaze of the first radiology tech. "This is the first mammogram they have on file for you, so don't be alarmed if they want more images," she says. "They just want to get to know your body."

Then a few days after that first mammogram, in a different clinic, yet another face. A different tech takes more detailed images. Her dark eyebrows pull together; her hair is long and straight and streaked with fuchsia. She crouches and peers up at me from underneath the machine, gazing intently at the smooth white arc of my left breast, while she aligns plates for the third image. Without cheer in her voice, she increases the pressure, asking, "You still okay?" and listening for my "Yep, I'm fine" before twisting the knob again. And again.

An hour after those follow-up images—as I tell myself, *nothing to be concerned about, they just want to get to know my body*—another young woman, unblinking, rubs an ultrasound wand over the gel on my left breast, first in circles, then in rows, increasing pressure, holding still in one spot, in another. She chews slightly on the inside of her cheek, accenting the heart shape of her face, but otherwise shows no expression.

When she's done, she hands me a towel, her voice kind. "The results will go back to your family doc, probably by..." She consults a chart. "Maybe tomorrow. Or no, it's a holiday. Monday for sure. I know you must be worried."

I must be worried? I wipe myself with the towel automatically and find that yes, I have been worried. My wee-hour concerns have shifted focus, from general life insults to the state of my left breast, without my conscious awareness. But I'm aware of worry now.

I leave the clinic and stop at the grocery store. There, I consult my list and put lettuce and carrots and milk into a basket. As I head toward the checkout, I think, "Who the fuck am I kidding?" and buy ice cream on a two-for-one special, my first taste in more than a year.

A few days after the follow-up images, still the holiday weekend, still waiting for results, I am restless. Most of the ice cream has disappeared, and I'm done with it anyway. I want to nurture myself with real food. I want to connect with my mother and my sister, as two or three of us together made devilled eggs in eight or ten different kitchens throughout the past fifty years.

I crack eggs, thinking of all of those new faces that are now part of my medical history. And I see still other faces: those of the children I didn't have. The colourful covers of the books I haven't yet written. And the faces of my mother, my sister.

* O *

* Secrets for the Best Devilled Egg Filling *

Separate yolks from whites. {You may also add whites that tore during peeling or that are otherwise imperfect.}

Using two knives {a pastry cutter : a fork} cut yolks into smaller-than-pea-sized pieces.

Into the yolks, mix real mayonnaise {use Miracle Whip : never use Miracle Whip}, mustard {dry mustard, hand-ground : yellow hot dog mustard : coarse brown deli mustard : honey-mustard : whatever is in your fridge}, salt and pepper {yes, salt, even if you're cutting out salt, the filling must have salt, also pepper : watch the salt and use only white pepper, so you get the flavour; black looks gross, like bug bits}, and a splash of a form of vinegar {dill pickle juice : sweet pickle juice : just add pickle relish : pickle relish makes it no different from egg salad : not pickle juice, just a splash of white vinegar : use prepared mustard and skip this} to taste {forget vinegar}. Experiment: {never} add curry!

Mix filling until it holds together. Then {using a small spoon : using an icing tube with a fancy cake-decorating tip : seriously?} fill the bowl of each egg white with approximately two teaspoons of filling.

Garnish as desired {with a sprinkle of paprika : with a slice of pimento-stuffed green olive or sweet gherkin : with a jalapeño slice : with a slice of black olive : with a tiny parsley leaf : seriously?}.

* o *

Nulliparous: Being nulliparous, as I am—not bringing forth a child, making that choice once, twice, monthly throughout decades—increases my risk of developing both ovarian and breast cancer. More consequences I didn't foresee.

Still, I've never regretted my choice. If could backtrack along my life's path, I wouldn't choose differently. But what if it had never been my choice to make? What if I'd wanted children and been unable to get pregnant? How unfair that would feel.

* o *

Crunchity-crunchity-crunch.

I roll the hard-boiled eggs against the sink surfaces and between my hands. I break the inner membrane and slide off the attached pieces of shell. I rinse the egg to remove those last, tiny, diamond-sharp bits.

Before I slice each egg open, I hold it in my palm.

I marvel at how white and smooth the eggs are, like my left breast in those dim rooms, where the only light came from a computer screen. The screen on which I glimpsed spotty images, like constellations spinning around a bright spot in the centre of my left breast.

Constellations are pictures from the past—the star twinkles actually occurred thousands of years ago. Winking at me from that computer screen was a picture from my own past—my history, and my family history. The consequences of decisions I'd made in my 20,000-plus days of living, combined with the effects of innumerable perfect and imperfect cell divisions and reproductions, after one ovum and one spermatozoon found each other decades ago.

I roll each peeled, damp egg on the towel before slicing it open. Yolks accumulate in the red bowl. I put each empty half onto a glass plate made especially for devilled eggs—eighteen ovals around the edge, with room for six or eight halves bunched in the plate's centre.

The day after I make the devilled eggs, I learn that I'm scheduled for a biopsy to investigate that bright spot in my left breast. *They're just getting to know your body* has lost all comfort for me. So I reframe my worry yet again: *Better to know, right? Information is power!*

Just before the biopsy, they take yet another set of still-more-powerful images. These images convince the radiologist that the bright spot is simply my own tissue. I'll have another mammogram in six months. I can relax until then. My sleep will improve.

But as I stir the filling that day I'm making eggs and thinking of faces, I don't know that I'll need a biopsy, or that I won't need one after all.

That day, I simply do the job. I cut up egg yolks; I sprinkle salt and pepper; I add mustard and mayonnaise. Nine years ago, I made devilled eggs for my wedding reception, while my sister kibitzed and commented on my filling choices. Both of us missed our mother that day. Round and round: my mother, my sister, and me. My stir-spoon traces the interior face of the bowl and I, too, circle, from breast to ovaries.

It comes back to eggs—all the eggs my ovaries have held and released. My ovaries float around in my abdomen, unable as always to tell me directly how they're doing. Since my hysterectomy they've been unable even to send me messages through the thickening and release of uterine lining. But I've never wondered what they were up to, not until my recent wakeful, sweaty nights. If they ever functioned, which I can't automatically assume, are they still going strong? Or are they finally tired?

I dip my pinkie into the bowl to taste the filling. After another sprinkle of salt and a final stir to mix it in, I wash my hands. I think of my family history and all its dead ends. And me, my dead beginnings. My ovaries, unused. My no-varies.

I scoop filling into a teaspoon and, with my forefinger, push it into the round cavity in each white oval, working my way around the plate. I have no need for garnish. This is my last step—how I do it, whether or not I'm doing it right.

18

ATOMIC TANGERINE

I. Remember Me

Imagine a late-September Saturday, the sun a plump golden grapefruit in a sky finally clear of summer's humid haze. Classes at Oklahoma State University would have started a month before. Call it Parents' Weekend, in 1979, or '85, or '88.

Visitors would clog the usually empty sidewalks of downtown Stillwater, Oklahoma. As Mom and I, intent on some unavoidable errand, threaded between people, he—inevitably a man—would step in front of her.

"Dr. Agnew, do you remember me?" A challenge.

And, beside me, I'd feel my mother sag.

I'd glare at the man with all the force my teenaged or twenty-something self could muster. His short-sleeved plaid cotton shirt with khakis or twill slacks or crease-pressed denim. His round or long face with thinning hair, a wide smile, ruddy cheeks. After OSU, he'd have gone on to sell insurance, or cattle, or houses. He was in town this weekend because his little brother, or maybe a son or daughter, was a student.

An innocuous-seeming question. But he was just so *sure* of his cleverness. *Do you remember me?*

"Um," my mother would say. "Well…" Mom had started teaching at OSU in 1948.

He'd prompt her: "Algebra, in 1960—no wait, must have been '71. Or maybe '72."

"Ah," Mom would answer. "I see. Sorry, I can't quite…." Algebra classes met in 500-seat auditoriums.

Finally, he'd say his name—Phil, Sonny, C.W., Gary—then add, "You gave me a D." Or, less often, "I told my little brother to try to get in your section," or "That was the class I worked hardest at."

Even less often: "Thank you!"

Sometimes small talk would come next—what he was up to now.

"Oh, how interesting," Mom would say, or "Good for you!" He'd never ask about her teaching, her research, her interests.

After he let us walk on, lamentation.

"How many students does he imagine I had in 1971, anyway?" she'd say. "How many students have I taught, before or since?"

A few steps later, "And I didn't 'give him' a D. He earned it."

Then she'd tell me, "Don't ever do that. Always say *your* name first."

I'd commiserate and soothe. It was an old story—she wasn't good with names. She'd said so, always. Ever since I could remember.

II. Morning Inventory

Three or four decades later, 1800 kilometres north, it's an early June morning. At 4:00 a.m., the sky lightens from navy blue through plums, fuchsias, and pinks into peach and light green and finally gold. The sun breaks the horizon well before 6:00, sending yellow- orange light streaming through our bedroom window. Reflections off Lake Superior ripple across the ceiling. I squint at the sun and roll over, trying to wrap sleep around me again.

In six months, you'll crave this light, this life around you. I force myself out of bed. June mornings are still cool enough to enjoy coffee warm, without ice. I take my mug onto the deck. A breeze off the lake touches my cheek. The ravens nesting on the cliff beside the house, screened from view by tall birch and spruce trees, cronk and trill a liquid greeting to the morning. I listen to the squirrels scolding—am I bothering them?—in the red pines.

The white-throated sparrow sings its disconcertingly cheerful "hard times in Canada, Canada," while chickadees and nuthatches buzz through the spruce and balsam firs. A pileated woodpecker shrieks and then drills a tattoo high in a dead birch. The kingfisher ratchets his way along the shoreline beside the two-track path leading to my family's camp.

Shading my eyes with my free hand, I look over the bay to birds at rest and in flight, and I whisper the names I'm learning, those of my morning companions on the water. "Geese, gulls, mallards, cormorants, mergansers." It is a chant without a regular refrain: "Goldeneye, mergansers, gulls, geese." I hope for loons. Some mornings, an eagle hunts high above us, harassed by crows and gulls.

III. Nothing Much

My mother excelled at so many things: research, teaching, service. At challenging colleagues as well as students. At finding interesting and useful mathematics problems to solve—and solving them. At thinking about teaching methods, finding grants to carry out her ideas, connecting theory with reality.

At home, she prized efficiency over creativity. Yet for decades, she cooked Sunday dinners for a family of seven, plus guests. She hosted the annual Christmas party for all of the church's women's groups.

For fun, she read, mostly mysteries—Erle Stanley Gardner until she discovered Ngaio Marsh and P.D. James. She crocheted afghans. An avid sports fan, she followed OSU wrestling matches and baseball/football/basketball games. She enjoyed university plays and concerts.

I know these things about her—I was often there, too—but I can't remember conversations. I remember recurring events, like former students stopping us and their demands to be remembered, but not specific incidents.

Sometimes I get glimpses. I see Mom in her chair at the end of the dining room table at our Oklahoma home, her fingers tapping her china coffee mug. Or in the kitchen, wrestling a flat-bottomed pan, heavy with a roasted turkey.

From the white counters and yellow appliances in the kitchen in Oklahoma, I flash to the small yellow camp on Lake Superior. There, she stands in dungarees and sweatshirt at the wood stove under the low, slanting ceiling. She pokes at the fire before adding another birch split, while oatmeal bubbles in a saucepan.

Or outdoors, in her black-and-white swimsuit that sets off her steel-grey hair, stepping gingerly off the rocks into the frigid water and making her way over the sand until the water laps at her waist. Then she pushes off but holds her head out of the water for lopsided, scissor-kicked breaststrokes in the sun-dappled bay.

She carries pails of water from the lake, launches the rowboat, sits on a tree stump to watch the lake wake up.

But in most of these pictures, I can't quite hear her laugh. I can't recall a time when she said something meaningful to me, or I said anything in particular to her.

In those days, I would have said I was paying attention, but I wasn't. I didn't know I needed to. I didn't know how much I'd want to remember those "nothing much" moments. I thought I'd always have them—that she'd always be here. Here with me. Here at the lake.

IV. Knowing Names

This summer morning on my deck is June 22. This part of the Lake Superior shoreline is the territory of the Anishinaabe peoples, as defined more than 150 years ago in the Robinson Superior Treaty of 1850. Yesterday, members of the Fort William First Nation led celebrations in Thunder Bay with dancing and drums, songs and chants, traditions and reverence and joy.

Twenty kilometres up the shoreline, I watch the lake wake up and wonder about the Indigenous people who knew the marshy waterfront in front of me, whether rice once grew wild among its grasses, whether they caught the sturgeon that return to lay eggs in years when the water is shallow. I wonder who loved the small protected bay to my right, not marshy at all, where a pebble-sand beach slopes gradually into the bone-chilling water on golden-orange mornings, sheltered from the breeze by the tall basalt-and-granite cliff where eagles nest.

Later, I'll brave the chilly water, but just now, beyond the thirty-foot spruce tree that towers between my deck and the water, a bird laughs. It's not a raven—the sound is more gurgle than cronk, and coming from the water. I walk along the deck for a better view, but tall grasses obscure the shoreline. Sound travels over water, so the call could have come from one of many distant black spots far out in the bay. As I head indoors for my second cup of coffee, I look up. A black bird approaches from the right to circle the house, and I glimpse its wildly beating wings as it streaks past. A cormorant.

I name it. I know it.

That's the point of my inventory, to call everyone by name. If I know them—not only birds, but rocks and trees and animals of all kinds—surely they also know me. And if they know me, then I belong here, too.

V. BLACK+BIRD

In my forties, almost five years after my mother died, I moved from Colorado to the north shore of Lake Superior. To ground myself in my new-yet-decades-familiar home, to help nurture and honour my roots, I have learned names of animals and plants.

And these names remind me of Eric, my Deaf American Sign Language teacher, back in Colorado. I took ASL classes after my mother died. I needed to learn something new: new ideas, a new language for the new world that no longer held my mother. As we learned signs for various animals, I asked how to sign "raven." Eric showed me: the sign for BLACK and then the sign for BIRD, written as BLACK+BIRD.

I said, "But a raven isn't the same as a blackbird or crow."

Eric said, "Then fingerspell it": with the alphabet, specify R-A-V-E-N or C-R-O-W. After I nodded to show I understood, he drew his eyebrows together. "Why do hearing people always want to limit something by giving it a label?"

I said again, "But crows and blackbirds are different. Using different names shows respect."

He said, "Deaf people focus on what birds *do*. We don't pretend to know who they are."

I sat back. It was my first direct experience of how language can shape the ways you think and live, and thus your whole world.

I've not forgotten that conversation with Eric, one of many. As I've learned names, I've also tried to learn what animals and plants do. I note where cormorants flock on late-summer mornings and how desperate they look in flight. I observe which rocks on the cliff the ferns cling to in their cascades, and when the moss transitions from cushioning my steps to crunching beneath them. I watch the relentless focus with which the lynx hunts snowshoe hares in early-spring twilights, how autumn storms scud across the sky to make and remake the beach, how deer hooves leave heart shapes in the snow.

But never mind what animals and plants do—what am *I* doing? Why bother with the names, with all this observation?

Honestly? I don't know. Maybe I deserve any scolding a squirrel wants to dish out on a summer morning.

Maybe I'm assembling a child's jigsaw puzzle—a landscape. The background horizon, where lake meets sky, is painted on thick wood, and each element lifts out in one piece. Dozens of bird-shaped pieces would include all the waterfowl as well as ravens and crows, blue and grey jays, and several different woodpeckers. For trees: spruce and balsam fir, birch and poplar, and many shrubbier types, like Manitoba "moose" maple and tag alder. I'd add puzzle pieces for the bunchberries, wild strawberries, clover, and grasses underfoot, and the purple and yellow wildflowers—asters, wild peas, bluebells, harebells, and thistles; oxeyes, butter-and-eggs, and dandelions. And animals: black bears, snowshoe hares, chipmunks, squirrels of different colours, does and fawns, a buck or two. A fox. At least one lynx, and perhaps a bobcat. Voles and mice, muskrats and otters.

I point to these puzzle pieces and say their names, and I feel proud. When I fit pieces into place, I feel accomplished, as if assembling the puzzle means something. As if I somehow had a hand in making the physical landscape.

How very Western, hearing culture, hierarchical, patriarchal. I know your name, therefore, I know you. I add you to a list or put you in a box, and you're mine—I own you.

VI. Promised Land

My grandmother liked to name things. She christened the family's first camp Cainaan, a play on LeCaine, the family name, and the biblical concept of "the promised land," because it was promised to our family as the Old Testament's Canaan was promised to the Israelites. In our case, it was a mining company, a lesser deity, that made the promise. The company, which had claimed land along Lake Superior for exploration, had assured people who built temporary camp structures that they'd have the first chance to buy someday. As the years passed, Cainaan came to refer both to the camp structure and to the land where it stood.

Grandma eventually named the second, larger camp Idyllwylde. My parents spelled it Idlewild, perhaps in quiet judgment of the romantic extravagance of "idyll." My siblings and I vary in our spelling choices.

I wonder what Grandma would call the 1980s-era house where Roy and I live. We haven't named it, instead labelling it with the word we raise in celebration as we pass under the birch that arches over our twisting driveway: Home.

Our names, all names, are a form of shorthand, a finger pointing to *this* spot *here*, not *that* one *there*. This place exists; it has a name. When we're no longer there, we can still name it.

On sunny summer mornings, walking the path to Cainaan or searching beaches for scoured-smooth bits of glass, I sometimes wonder what of this place my mother remembered in that last year, when she had lost so much of herself. She had loved Cainaan for seventy-five years by then—were the place and its name as deeply embedded in her as her own name was?

Sometimes I wonder what this place remembers of my mother. The woodshed behind Cainaan still has a board set up as a desk in one corner. She wrote her dissertation there in 1940. My grandfather gave Cainaan to her as a graduation present in 1941, before she married. During the Second World War, when she researched nuclear equations in Ottawa and Montreal, she still spent time at Cainaan. After she settled in Oklahoma, she brought the family up to Cainaan every summer, even if we could stay only three weeks, ten days, a week.

In the 1940s, my parents were the first to paint Cainaan yellow, with green trim and roofing paper. Grandma had always favoured a rich, warm reddish-brown, which we grandchildren occasionally found in traces under the repainted window trim and christened "Grandma Orange."

A few summers ago, my husband and I again painted the camp's exterior. The trim became a deep plum, to complement the new brown roofing paper. And I chose a bright shade of gold for the walls. Both my mother's war work and Grandma Orange echo in the colour's name—Atomic Tangerine. In this small way, I make sure they are remembered here.

VII. C-H-O-R-T-L-E, M-A-P-L-E

All summer, a raven greets us with its croaking laugh from the nest on the cliff, and we say, "Hi, Chortle," but it might be a different bird each time, and it certainly doesn't call itself "Chortle" or even "raven."

I can distinguish specific trees—they don't move, so the poplar at the edge of the driveway is always the same poplar—but I don't know each tree as an individual. I don't know how their lives have been shaped by their specific locations, as my life has been.

Except in the case of one maple tree. My husband brought it from a lawn in southern Ontario and planted it on the lake side of the house. In late September, its leaves don't redden as they did in the south; they turn golden, tinged with orange, before dropping. I'm no arborist, so I'm not sure why, but it lives at *this* place, *here*. It's cool for maples at our latitude, and our soil is full of sand and clay. Maybe those are reasons enough.

It comes back to this question: *So what?* Even if I could distinguish an individual chipmunk burrowing in our septic field or leaping among the pine branches, even if I could give its complete ancestry going as far back as my grandparents' time, what would that prove, and to whom?

VIII. Precision, Pervasiveness

As I take inventory of the natural world around me, the names I'm learning are less precise than I anticipated.

For example, "robin" refers to different birds in English-speaking Europe, North America, and Australia, and the "red breast" of folk songs is orange in North America.

Amethyst—Ontario's provincial gemstone, mined a few kilometres from our home—is only one colour variant of quartz, which ranges from black-purple through shades of violet, lavender, and pink to white. Quartz nuggets are common on our beach, and some bear veins that shine a soft lilac.

For someone who only recently learned that "rocks" and "minerals" are different things, who learned the names of semi-precious gems from jewellery ads, it's disconcerting to see the fluidity of what I think I know and to sense the magnitude of what I have yet to learn.

Other examples of our human fascination with names are as numerous as the rocks (or minerals) underfoot. In religion, from A to Z: Adam of the Judeo-Christian tradition assigns names to the animals; Zoroastrians have 101 names for Ahura Mazda. In fairy tales: if the miller's (usually unnamed) daughter can't guess Rumpelstiltskin's name, he'll take her firstborn child.

And we understand that names have power. In medicine, the World Health Organization recently suggested naming all new diseases and infections with general descriptive terms—the symptoms or the pathogen, such as respiratory disease or coronavirus. Illnesses named with terms of geography (Spanish flu), animal species (bird flu), or people (Alzheimer's) can provoke backlash: unnecessary trade restrictions, needless slaughter of food animals, or unfairly unpleasant associations with a name.

IX. Boating Companions

My mother pulls one oar and pushes the other, and the aluminum rowboat, which the family named the *Trudi-Jeanne*, spins to point toward the islands in the bay. She leans forward and then back, and the boat skims over the water's surface.

Who kept my mother company when she rowed? Did she think of her parents, my uncle and aunt? Or perhaps other people who'd been important in her life. Her advisor at Harvard in the 1930s, G. D. Birkhoff, who took her on reluctantly because the other female student he'd advised had left mathematics to marry and have five children. Mom loved to tell that story and wait for people to realize that she'd married and had five kids, too—but she hadn't left mathematics, any more than she'd really left behind this camp at the lake.

When I row to the island, I notice gulls, cormorants, and loons. I watch the world, its sun and sky and waves. I monitor the wind direction and strength. I name the colours of the water, lichens, rock: mallard green, near-neon orange, charcoal grey.

I watch the camp wink at me through birches from the shoreline. I think about the property tax my family has paid for decades, the insurance we have carried—the formal ceremonies of my culture's ownership that let me enjoy the birds and rocks around me but have nothing to do with them. As the lake breathes beneath me, I mull over words and phrases: *traditional territory, family property, treaty peoples. Fairness, equity. Owning, belonging.*

I wonder whether my husband watches through binoculars to be sure I'm safe. I wish my sister were here, my brothers with their families. My parents—my mother.

X. Namesakes, Squared

In many cultures, names echo through generations. Children are given the same name as an adult—usually a relative. These children—namesakes—are thought to have personalities similar to the adult for whom they're named.

When my mother was born in 1917, thirty-one girls born in Ontario that year were also named "Jeanne." She was named for my maternal great-grandmother, Jane. But "Jane LeCaine" didn't please my grandmother's ear. Hence Jeanne.

The year my mother turned eighty, another name—"Alzheimer's disease"—entered our family lexicon. In the years before her illness, my mother wrote textbooks and collected beautiful stamps and had her hair done at a beauty salon on Fridays or Saturdays so that her hair would be presentable for church on Sunday. She advised students, organized meetings of professional mathematics societies, and led Cub Scout dens; she monitored piano practice, drove carpools, and sat through dozens of heats of 11-12 girls' 200 IM at swim meets, winter and summer.

Her longed-for first child, a son, died after eleven hours of struggled breathing. As the five of us surviving siblings appeared, she was thrilled to hear us call her "Mom," "Mommy," "Mother." Yet beyond that role, she remained "Jeanne." She dreamed and wrote and solved math problems and taught and laughed and cried.

I wish I could better remember my pre-disease mother—my unimpaired mother. But I carry part of her with me always: Jeanne is my middle name.

Before my father died, he hadn't drifted as far away as my mother had—in fact, he had come closer to us. Now, as I navigate politics and citizenship in two countries, I often wish I could ask for his historical perspective. I think of him with a mixture of exasperation and fondness every time I dither over a decision or yell at a news announcer on television. I'm proud to carry his last name.

XI. Someday, Always

Friends sometimes ask whether I'm afraid I'll get Alzheimer's too. It's a fair question. With my grandmother's dementia, it's a large part of our family's story.

I say, "Of course." And I suppose I am—I'm wary, at least. Learning, observing, and taking inventory are just a few of the ways I keep challenging my brain.

But I'm also not afraid, because my mother and I are different people, and I can't see very far into the future. At this moment, I live in *this* place, *here*, through long winter nights lit by the aurora borealis as well as summer evenings when the twilight lingers late. I hope to live here always, whatever "always" means.

I like to think about "always," the length of time my mother remained Jeanne. But because I can't see the future, I think backwards.

I set aside the years of my lifetime, my whole family—my siblings and me, my mother and father, and before them, my grandparents. Set aside the mining companies and governments, the Europeans, French and English. Even the Indigenous families among us, who know themselves and this region by different names. Thousands of years of ancestors embraced this landscape, made tools at a site just a kilometre away (as the raven flies), knew its birds and animals and trees. They painted orange-red figures on cliff faces at the other end of this inland sea, celebrated the sun's rising and setting, and told stories under midwinter's aurora borealis.

And yet, before any of us, before any humans, this land once existed. She will endure long after we're gone. She names many generations of humans in her inventory. She teaches me about so many things, including eternity and love, and I'm grateful. And although I can't own her, not really, I do belong to her for always, as I hope she does, for my always, to me.

19

HOURS OF DAYLIGHT (II)

This is a story about what (doesn't) change.
After my mother died I found myself missing her—all of her—again. And I knew that Dad missed her more, and more of her, than I could comprehend. Our sadness drew us together. I developed a new respect for Dad's routines—even his index cards and ballpoint pens—as I watched them help him befriend grief and carry on for the seven years until his last illness.

***

This is a story of waiting, and of hope.
Alzheimer's disease is still out there. Perhaps it's not only *out there* but also *in here*, quietly growing in my own brain. Our family has escaped the disease's known genetic markers, but we're still at increased risk. Mom's mother also showed signs of senile dementia in the 1950s.

Periodically, I look into the ways people with Alzheimer's can live. In a Colorado residence, I see how something as simple as the building's design—a square around an open-air courtyard—allows people to wander and even go outdoors in safety. I watch the activities leader involve the laughing, cheerful residents in daily exercise. She and I sit in silence in the parlour with a grief-stricken daughter, holding an understanding place for her pain.

Terms change, and with them, so does my perspective. "Alzheimer patients" become "people with Alzheimer's"—people first. Privacy laws in both Canada and the U.S. have strengthened the "nothing about us without us" elements of health care.

"Caregivers" become "care partners," and I remember how my mother's face brightened when she saw my father in the nursing home—I hope he saw it, too, and felt her love for him. I think of the morning of Mom's funeral, when Dad slipped out onto the porch with a small sewing kit she had prepared years before, when she also showed him how she washed his socks and underwear. Sue and I saw him from the living room but let him sit alone, away from the rest of us but communing with Mom, to sew a button on his jacket.

I try to remember the value, to research, of negative results. Even when you want to know what something *is*, sometimes knowing what it *isn't* can be helpful. Some twenty years after my mother's "probable" diagnosis, researchers know a lot more about what the Alzheimer's disease process isn't.

Through the years, Alzheimer's stays in the news. On the cover of the January/February 2011 of *Discover*, a line trumpeted "Medicine: Alzheimer's Cure." I grabbed the magazine from the dining room table and flipped through the pages, scanning madly. Finally, the story: "Early Diagnosis for Alzheimer's."

Early diagnosis. Oh.

Almost fourteen years after reading my mother's Christmas card, I slumped into a chair at a different kitchen table to read about the new tools that make it possible for doctors to diagnose Alzheimer's with 90 percent or greater accuracy.

Important results, yes. But not a cure.

We're all still waiting for that.

* * *

This is the story of an oblate spheroid spinning on its axis and orbiting the sun.

My parents have both been gone for years. I know that only because I remind myself. Sometimes it seems as if they could still be living in the house in Oklahoma. But someone else sleeps in those upstairs bedrooms now—a lovely young family, the mother a former mathematics graduate student and the father an engineer; in my father's study, they and their children film science and art videos and post them to YouTube.

One April, my siblings and I rendezvous in Oklahoma for the first time in the decade since my father's death. My sister suggests we crash the Oklahoma State Mathematics Department awards ceremony, where every year, two students receive awards named for my mother. We aren't sure we'll know anyone—Mom's former young colleagues are now past retirement age.

But my sister and I recognize Jim Choike, who once dreamed up projects and grant applications with Mom around our dining room table. We ask him to explain the Hours of Daylight problem.

Dr. Choike says the problem was supplied by McDonnell Douglas. For their Mars Rover project, they needed to know whether it's possible to calculate the hours of daylight at any location on Earth knowing only its latitude and longitude and the day of the year.

Years ago, Mom's applied math students demonstrated that yes, it is possible to calculate the hours of daylight with only that information. But to come up with their solution, they had to make one simplification in their assumptions—that the Earth is a perfect sphere.

"And," Dr. Choike says, "as you know—"

The three of us say it together. "The Earth is an oblate spheroid." We laugh.

And blink back tears. Because now, only the story remains. Still, the story remains.

20

REVERBERATIONS

*"For the more haunted among us, only looking back
at the past can permit it finally to become past."*
–Mary Karr, *The Art of Memoir*

Roy comes in from mowing the grass. I meet him at the front door. While he removes his hat and bulbous ear protectors, I fidget, impatient with what I want to say.

"I would like to write about something other than my mother. In fact, I'd like to write about something other than dead people. You know, in general."

He pulls a handkerchief from his pocket and wipes sweat from his forehead. "Okay. So—do it."

I go outdoors to poke around on our ten acres. I wonder what else I could write about. I listen.

The sound of a landscape—its everyday murmurings, its "normal"—is its undersong.

I imagine our place on Lake Superior as silent, especially when I spend any time in a city of any size. But when I stop to listen, I learn otherwise.

Voices ring out in the big sandy bay—laughs and shouts from shivering children, standing waist-deep in chilly Lake Superior, splashing each other. They fling water drops into the air to flash in the sun, calling "Diamonds!" Other kids, in canoes or on rafts, dare each other to thread the obstacle course in the shallows where underwater boulders lurk, most often detected by a screeching impact of watercraft on rock.

Summer mornings, flocks of gulls and crows squabble endlessly. In summer's long twilight evenings, a lone duck's comical call: "Quack! Quack-quack! Quack!"

And the trains. The trains! The non-Indigenous experience of North America, maybe especially those in the central and western parts of the continent, seem inextricably tied to trains. Much has been written about their "lonesome" whistles and the dull, rhythmic drone of wheel on rail, transporting someone to a new life, new adventures. It's all very romantic.

We've heard trains, too, through the years. They arced around the lake on two sets of tracks at different times, the CP Line and the CN Line, both just out of sight beyond ridges or stands of trees. One line no longer has traffic and serves as a playground for ATVs and snow machines, but trains still make the circuit on the other, still blowing their whistles at crossings.

For generations, voices from my family have laughed here. The sounds of children playing don't necessarily pin down this location in time. The voices could be from the 1920s and '30s, the '50s and '60s, the '80s and '90s, or even the 20-teens, from my family alone.

Some evenings and mornings and random afternoons, as the weather and seasons permit, I walk the rock-and-sand beach in front of our smaller camp, thinking of nothing and everything. I pick up an interesting-looking rock.

In my ear, I hear my mother. "Remember when Uncle Allen came to visit?"

Allen, my father's brother, felt about rocks and geology the way my father did about U.S. presidents and American social history.

"Remember? How I'd show him the most beautiful rocks, something like this pink quartz one, or that interesting speckled one over there, and he'd look at it and say, 'Yes, that's very nice.' Then he'd pick up some ordinary rock, dull and brown, or even grey—the most boring thing on the beach! And he'd say, 'But look at this! Now this is really something, it's—' whatever it was."

As always when telling a story about how someone else enjoyed this place, she laughs, and I smile.

An echo is a single sound that runs into something that sends the sound wave back toward its origin. A reverberation is more complicated—several sounds echo, or one sound echoes several times. The sound waves cross each other, interacting as they go.

But for echoes and reverberations to work as defined, time must move forward. Meanwhile, philosophers say that "eternity" doesn't mean "forever," as the rest of us think. Instead, it refers to time that stands outside our experience of past, present, and future.

Some physicists (notably Einstein) propose some version of this statement: all time exists now. The mathematics of their argument is too advanced for me to follow.

While I meander the beach, surrounded by lake whispers, I sometimes feel a little of what Einstein might have meant, or perhaps the philosopher's eternity.

There, I can sit on a log and close my eyes, and I'm three years old again, emptying a blue plastic pail of sand onto the beach, or with my cousin, kneeling beside the dishpan full of water to sail bits of wood we christen "boats." I can be twelve and paddling the yellow canoe, adopted by our crew after it was cast ashore by a lake storm one spring. Or in my thirties, escaping the shore and my troubles in the rowboat while someone else distracts my mother so that her agitation, brought on by Alzheimer's, is directed elsewhere. Or in my mid-forties, when I stare at the lake and inhale, and I finally admit that the marriage I don't want to return to after my vacation is far less real to me than my relationship with this beach, this place, this lake.

Today, any day, I walk along the beach toward the break in the trees where we string the water line in the summer. From under the alder, I'll pick up a beaver-chewed poplar branch and think, "Was this here last time?" I'll find deep pointed tracks between the grasses and the water and wonder when the deer came through—a few minutes ago, or a few days? I'll shake the sand off a dirty white plastic bucket, one I don't recognize, and fret, hoping it was tossed on the beach by the lake, not a human trespasser. As I walk home, I'll pick up birch branches that fell onto the path just in the hour since I walked the other direction.

At least that's when I think they fell. Perhaps they were there before—perhaps they were there all along, perhaps they're always there. Just as all the versions of myself are still there on the log and the water and the beach and the path, even versions I have not yet become.

The lake plays the biggest role in our place's undersong. We hear its quiet murmurs and shushes most often early in the morning or as evening falls. In blips and flups, the lake exhales and inhales around rocks at the shoreline. Gradually, a quiet lake fades from centre stage and gives lead roles to others: the wind swirls through birch and poplar leaves, sparrows twitter among the shrubby alder and Manitoba maple, gulls complain and ravens converse, an eagle screams like sheet metal shredding.

Other days, the lake demands its due. Changeable weather causes choppy waves that slap-smack a rowboat's side and send canoes swaying fore-and-aft, side-to-side. Wind and pressure out on what my mother called the "big lake," beyond the Sibley peninsula, create waves in a long rolling surf. They travel kilometres through the water along Thunder Bay to fling themselves on the rocky cliffs of islands and outcrops, and up the shore of sloping beaches like ours. They boom and crash, like a stadium full of human voices cheering or jeering.

The waves have been here as long as the lake has—which is to say, longer than anyone I know or have known, living or dead.

I started writing about my mother after her Alzheimer's diagnosis, long after we knew something was wrong. I received a Christmas card from her, full of gibberish, and couldn't pretend any longer. That holiday, I began writing what I saw.

My father died seven years after my mother, and as my siblings and I went through their house in Oklahoma, everything—every paper, every box—related to Mom, the land in Canada, or her side of the family was sent back north with me. And since both of my parents lived through the Depression and spent their adult lives far away from their parents, they prized letters highly and kept them.

I haven't read all the letters my mother exchanged with her own mother, but one afternoon, searching boxes to see if I'd missed any legal documents relating to our property, I noticed a letter from Grandma that Mom had set aside. Dated 1957, it's a thank-you note for the Christmas parcel my mother had sent. In it, my grandmother describes how she believes that the actors on television are aware of her and look for her as they perform. Later in the letter, she mentions a phone call from Mom's sister Allison, and talking with Bill—giving his last name in parentheses and explaining that Bill was Allison's husband.

Mom, of course, would have known that.

What must she have felt when she read these pages, when Grandma's handwriting in fountain pen had not yet faded?

I've known for years that Grandma had "hardening of the arteries" and died in 1965 after many years in a hospital. I remember visiting Grandma there. I remember how much it upset my mother when Grandma didn't know her.

But until I saw that letter, set apart from other bundles, I didn't know that Mom had received a Christmas letter of her own. I didn't understand that those years of Grandma's growing illness had been, for her, as treacherous and difficult as the years of her decline were for me.

As the years accumulate between my "now" and my mother's death, my experience of time puzzles me. How can things that happened long ago feel so present? My memories run together.

My mother wades into the clear, chilly water to dip and fill a metal bucket, far enough from shore to reduce the amount of sand she'll scoop up.

A rock spins and twists in an arc across the water's surface, the thrower a sibling, my mother or uncle, a niece or nephew or grandson or cousin, my husband or me.

The black stone of the flat outcrop warms my back, the sunlight behind my eyelids orange-hot, while the breeze from the water brings gooseflesh to my bare arms and legs. I have nearly six decades' worth of this experience, one from every summer I came here and at least one from every year I've lived here, when the level of the lake water is low enough that the flat rock peeks out of the water.

Through the decade I've lived here year-round and full-time, we've made changes. We've torn up and replaced the leaking roof at the smaller camp, adding a layer of plywood under the tarpaper and roofing paper. The house where I live with Roy also has a new roof. Both roofs still leak near the chimneys, when the rain is persistent and the wind is right. Or wrong.

The forward march of time brings other changes. My sister retires and spends more time at Idyllwylde, again altering the rhythms of our summers together. My brothers have grandchildren—new toddlers to play on the beach, to collect rocks and bits of birchbark and balsam branches as "specimens."

Other things don't change as much. I often hear my mother's voice in my ear, and not only when I'm remembering a story she used to tell. I have a vivid sense memory of her voice from my phone's answering machine, saying, "Marion, this is your mother." Similarly, I can hear my father's voice from his last months calling me "daughter dear," a real treat.

Through recent years, I have become increasingly estranged from sleep and often wake in the night. Sometimes I'm restless enough to get up and read; other nights, I escape Roy's snores in the guest bedroom, where I listen to the noises of the house and the outdoor sounds from a window in a different part of the house. I hear a train groaning as it rounds the end of the bay and wait for its whistle, feeling smug. *Could anything be more cliché than lying alone in bed, hearing a train in the night?*

The sound doesn't grow any louder, and I notice that the chug is rhythmic. Eventually, I realize what I hear isn't the train at all—it's my own heartbeat in my ears. I feel foolish—like a living cliché.

When I was young and announced that I wanted to live here someday, my mother was right to warn me about winter. The cold can feel endless and brutal. But I love living here year-round, while other people retreat to homes in town, or in Florida.

As long as winter puts pink in my cheeks but doesn't yet slice my lungs, I walk outdoors, sometimes even as far as the beach.

On the way, I hear sounds of late autumn and winter, its ravens, its chickadees, its grosbeaks. I see evidence of passages: the hare flashes by on snowshoe feet, with the lynx padding silently, inevitably, behind. A fox tip-tip-tips past, leaving prints in a straight line. Winter always holds more sound than I anticipate, even though I know better. There's the unsound-sound of snow falling, like the silvery hum of insomniac nights. Some months, the lake lies frozen but not immobile. The lake ice cracks and groans in her sleep.

Then a ceaseless high-pitched whine starts up, a snow machine towing an ice house out onto the lake so someone can fish. I turn back toward home. As I near the house, its heating system kicks on, startling me with clangs and hisses—a sound that, from indoors, barely registers as a purring thrum. How loud these human sounds must be to the fox and hare and lynx and deer.

I dislike inflicting ourselves, our noise, on the rest of the world, but I wonder what makes sounds acceptable, or not. We are animals, too. We live here now, too.

Summer or winter or somewhere in between, when I'm outdoors I can hear sounds of our human life as if they're present. Voices of the lake, and rowboats. Letters rustling, beach rocks plunking, music, leaking roofs. The voices of people, children and adults, related to me and not, who mow and rake and prune and dig and cut, who nail and paint and scrape, who sweep and bake and roast and polish the stove, who connect water lines and empty the outhouse pails, who row and paddle and pole and swim and splash. Who dream, and plan, and pay. And love.

Perhaps somewhere, somewhen, my mother walks the beach and picks up a bit of granite or jasper, an agate, a piece of pink driftglass. Perhaps she thinks of me.

We, and our echoes and reverberations, for better and worse, are part of the undersong.

On another day in another season, I again say to Roy, "I'd really like to write about something else. Not my dead mother or my dead father. And no more dead dogs, either."

He looks up from his laptop. His voice is cheerful, encouraging. "Good luck with that."

ACKNOWLEDGEMENTS

One late-August Saturday morning, I fill my coffee mug and head downstairs to search for a photo in the file boxes under the pool table. In the first box, I find a few items my father saved.

I examine the daily devotion book, turned to May 7, 2000. Dad's annotation is in blue ballpoint: "we 2, Grace, ca. 6 pm." In the daily thought, "As long as I have breath, I will serve the Lord," he underlined "have breath." That day's prayer request was for persons in nursing homes, like Grace Living Center, where my mother died of pneumonia near midnight, just a few hours after my father's daily visit.

I next find a few pages of notes he scribbled on the night of her death. Who he'd called and when. For my mother's obituary, the dates she was in graduate school. Hymns and scripture readings that might be appropriate for her funeral service.

Underneath the notes lie other photos. Several show Mom in her reclining chair, clutching a bouquet of gladiolas. They were brought by a mathematics graduate student who stands beside her chair, formal and respectful in a straight skirt and buttoned blazer. She won an award bearing Mom's name.

And finally, a photo of them both—"We 2"—from Mom's birthday, just four days before her death, taken by the Grace staff.

As it happens, the first box also holds the photo on the cover of this book: young Jeanne, "from about the time I first knew her," Dad told me once.

I'm grateful that these artifacts exist. I'm also grateful to close the photo album, return it to its box, slide the box under the pool table, and leave my basement office to fill my coffee mug and dry my eyes.

This book has been touched by many writerly hands as it's come into being. In Colorado, John Calderazzo provided encouragement and helpful comments on what later became "Home." Poet and friend Veronica Patterson asked what I'd been up to, and her bright "Oh! What was that like?" led me to write about Fancy's funeral, which became "All I Can Say." Jill Talbot provided feedback on an early version of "Atomic Tangerine."

In Canada, Susan Goldberg and Rebekah Skochinski found innumerable gentle ways to say, "This is about your mother," even when I didn't want to hear it. Susan Olding provided mentorship and honest scrutiny exactly when I needed it. Through the years, I'm very grateful that individual pieces were selected or recognized by Clélie Rich, Kathy Page, Wayne Grady, Betsy Warland, Lynne van Leuven, Janine Tschuncky and Andris Taskans, and readers at various literary journals and anthologies. The dedicated team at Signature Editions helped the disparate parts of this manuscript become a more coherent whole.

I owe a debt to the local writing community, especially to those who have led the Northwestern Ontario Writers Workshop through the years. Kudos also to the Ontario Arts Council for its work in sustaining artists of all disciplines, especially its support of this work through its Creator and Recommender grants. I appreciate the regular encouragement, laughter, and commiseration I've shared with other writers: Marianne Jones and Maureen Nadin, Cathi Winslow and Jean E. Pendziwol, and those who know how to finish the phrase, "The first rule..."

I'm grateful to the Colorado Deaf community, especially Eric Fifer, for welcoming my desire to learn; I hope I have shown in this work the respect I feel for you all. Also, thank you to people with experience of Alzheimer's and dementia. Your voices matter. And I also appreciate my mother's mathematics students and colleagues. I could name many, but I will stop with two. Dr. William

Durand, Mom's first doctoral student, helped me remember other iterations of my mother in her time of illness. Dr. James Choike, her colleague, recently reminded me of her lasting influence.

Families are precious and complicated, and I'm grateful to those I've been a part of. Bob and the rest of the Whobodies, Mark and his clan—and now Bill and Marcio, plus Karen, Jacob, Isaac, and Daniel. For decades, Tricia McConnell has been my ardent supporter while also calling me on my dithering, the truest sign of family.

I appreciate the support and forbearance of my siblings, each of whom writes and makes music. Lee is a brave and tenderhearted activist. Hugh combines dreaming with a devotion to duty. Pete—who stopped being "mean, as usual" to me forty-five years ago—is a gentle, principled force for good with whom I enjoy exchanging notes about the writing life. Sue's creative energy blossoms in many areas—visual art and cooking as well as words and music—and I appreciate her ongoing companionship, especially her courage in mouse disposal.

Roy, my Mr. Knightley, has been my supporter and partner through many years of care and happiness. His generosity of spirit continues to humble me. In writing and in life, his any is all to me.

Working on this book, off and on, for the past twenty years has given me many gifts. I'm most grateful for the opportunity to spend time with both of my parents—Jeanne Starrett LeCaine Agnew and Theodore Lee Agnew, Jr—in times of joy as well as illness. May they be granted a safe lodging, a holy rest, and peace at the last.

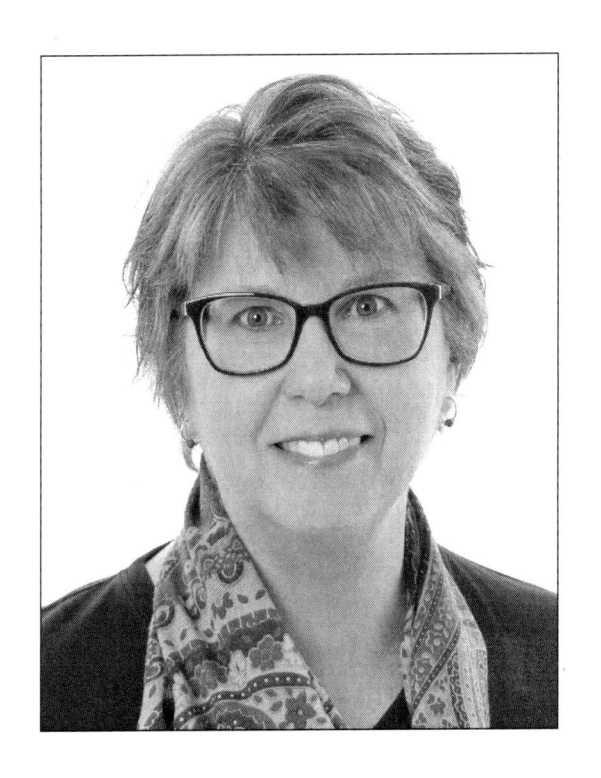

ABOUT THE AUTHOR

Marion Agnew's essays and short fiction have appeared in numerous magazines and literary journals, including *The Malahat Review*, *The New Quarterly*, *Atticus Review*, *The Walleye*, *The Grief Diaries*, and *Full Grown People*, as well as in the anthologies *Best Canadian Essays* 2012 and 2014. She has been shortlisted for the *Prairie Fire* contest as well as for a Pushcart Prize and Best of the Net. Originally from Oklahoma, she realized her dream of becoming a Canadian citizen and moving to the her family's summer property in the Canadian Shield, where she had spent the most magical summers of her childhood.

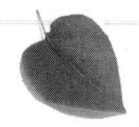

Eco-Audit
*Printing this book using Rolland Enviro 100 Book
instead of virgin fibres paper saved the following resources:*

Trees	Energy	Water	Air Emissions
3	6 GJ	1,000 L	222 kg